Hidden Food Allergies

Other Books by the Author

*New Developments in Allergy and How They Can Help You
Overcome Your Problem*

*Proven Steps To Overcome Airborne Allergens--
A Self Help Workbook*

Hidden Food Allergies

Stephen Astor, MD

⌐ AVERY PUBLISHING GROUP INC. ⌐

Garden City Park, New York

The medical and health procedures in this book are based on the training, personal experiences, and research of the author. Because each person and situation are unique, the editor and publisher urge the reader to check with a qualified health professional before using any procedure where there is any question as to its appropriateness.

The publisher does not advocate the use of any particular diet, but believes the information presented in this book should be available to the public.

Because there is always some risk involved, the author and publisher are not responsible for any adverse effects or consequences resulting from the use of any of the suggestions, preparations, or procedures in this book. Please do not use the book if you are unwilling to assume the risk. Feel free to consult a physician or other qualified health professional. It is a sign of wisdom, not cowardice, to seek a second or third opinion.

Cover design by Martin Hochberg and Rudy Shur
In-house editor Jacqueline Balla

Allergy-free recipes in Appendix C reprinted with permission of Ross Laboratories, Columbus, OH 43216, from "Cooking With *Isomil* Soy Protein Formula With Iron," © 1986 Ross Laboratories.

Reprinted with permission of Best Foods, A Unit of CPC North America, Englewood Cliffs, NJ.

Library of Congress Cataloging-in-Publication Data
Astor, Stephen H.
  Hidden food allergies.

  Includes index.
  1. Food allergy--Popular works.   2. Food allergy--
Diagnosis.   I. Title.
RC596.A8   1988   616.97'5   87-35124
ISBN 0-89529-369-2

Printed in the United States of America

10 9 8 7 6 5 4 3 2 1

Contents

This book is dedicated to my three favorite people—
Merry, Beth, and Jeff

Acknowledgements

I wish to acknowledge and thank the following for their suggestions during the writing of this book—Bettie J. Brigman, R.D.; Vera Fritz, M.P.H., R.D.; Susan Daglish, B.A.; and my editor, Jacqueline Balla.

Preface

There are two secrets to success in treating food allergy. The first is learning whether you do, in fact, suffer from food allergy. The second is discovering which food you are allergic to.

Hidden Food Allergies will teach you a step-by-step method of uncovering possible food allergy. The technique described has been proven successful in thousands of clinical cases.

When a patient is first told that a food may be responsible for his symptoms, he often protests, "But it can't be food because I've eaten the same things for years." On the contrary. A person is more likely to become sensitive to a food he has consumed over a long period of time than a food he rarely eats. The human body must be exposed to a substance in order to become sensitized to it. The greater the exposure, the greater the chance of allergic susceptibility.

No one is born with all the allergies that he may eventually experience. Nor can a person count on the fact that if he has not developed food allergy by the time he is a certain age, he is then safe. There is no "magic age" at which the human body becomes immune to allergy, or to any other disease, for that matter.

Because repeated exposure is necessary in order to sensitize an individual, experiments such as those by Dr. Robert Hamburger at the University of California's San Diego Medical Center have had disappointing results. In Dr. Hamburger's study, women with allergies (or whose families had a strong history of allergy) were encouraged to breastfeed their infants in the hope of preventing allergy in their offspring. At the end of the study period, these infants were not 100% protected against allergy. When this poor outcome was analyzed, the explanation became obvious.

If a child is born with genes that make him susceptible to an allergic reaction to, say, milk products, then delaying the introduction of milk into the infant's diet by breastfeeding would merely postpone the allergy. Breastfeeding can delay an inevitable sensitization to foods, but will not prevent it. Furthermore, breastfeeding would have no influence on a baby's exposure to grass pollen, ragweed pollen, dust, mold, or the family dog, and could not prevent these allergies from developing. If a mother wishes to breastfeed, then, she should do so for a reason other than the hope of curing allergies in her offspring.

Sometimes it takes great imagination to realize that an illness or other health problem may be caused by food allergy. People are hung up on the fact that foods produce only rashes and gastrointestinal problems, and other possibilities seem absurd to them.

How can food produce a headache? How can food make one tired? How can food provoke asthma or arthritis?

The answers to these questions are no mystery. Every food substance is made up of many different chemicals. In addition, other chemicals are added during processing. Foods are further altered by cooking, freezing, and pasteurizing. These chemicals and altered food substances are found throughout nature. They are present in living organisms such as livestock, poultry, and fish. They can be found in plant material such as grains, vegetables, herbs, and fruits. And they exist in inorganic materials such as salts, preservatives, and flavorings.

We consume these substances for nourishment and even the treatment of disease. Once inside the body, they have various effects on our cells and tissues. Sometimes the effect is pleasant, like the wonderful taste of chocolate. Sometimes the substances cause burning, as do hot peppers. Foods such as beans often produce unwanted gas. Chemicals like caffeine can produce nervousness. Prunes may cause diarrhea by a direct action on the gastrointestinal tract. Cheeses containing *tyramine* can produce headaches by the way they affect the blood vessels. Last, but not least, is the allergic kind of reaction. It is this type of reaction that is the subject of this book.

There are two types of allergic reactions. Antibody allergy is one such reaction. It is due to the overproduction of a specific antibody. We produce five types of antibodies: IgE, IgG, IgM, IgD, and IgA. Certain individuals have an inherited tendency to produce excess amounts of the IgE type. These people develop an allergy. When excess antibody is present, there is an excess reaction. That is why doctors call allergy a *hypersen-sitivity*.

The interesting fact about such allergies is that your body cannot make IgE unless you have been sufficiently exposed to the food. That is why trained allergists are more suspicious of a food that someone eats regularly than a food that is new to his diet.

The other type of allergy is called cellular allergy. Instead of producing too much IgE antibody, the individual has over-reactive lymphocytes. When exposed to certain chemical agents and proteins, these cells become sensitized. Subsequently, when the substance enters the body, the cells react to get rid of the foreign material. This process of expelling foreign material causes the reaction we know as cellular allergy. It is one of the body's major weapons for rejecting transplanted organs.

Thus, contrary to popular belief, allergy is not a weakness or a deficiency of the body. Rather, it is an intense reaction due to excessive quantities of certain antibodies and overreactions of certain cells. Such antibodies and cells are found throughout the body, from the surface of the skin down to the deepest tissues. They are present in every nook and cranny. When we ingest foods, our bloodstream carries them to all parts of our system—to every organ and cell—where the foods can react with the excessive antibodies or the over-reactive cells.

So allergy can affect the brain, the lungs, the heart, the blood vessels, the joints, and the muscles. It can also produce a variety of symptoms. You are now ready to answer two critical questions: "Are *my* symptoms due to allergy?" and *"To what extent* are my symptoms due to allergy?"

1
Introducing Food Allergy and Its Symptoms

Marilyn was 37 years old. She had always been an active and busy woman, but suddenly found herself tiring very easily. She also had constant headaches. Her doctors kept telling her that there was nothing wrong. They sent her to a psychiatrist, but her family life was in perfect order—she had great kids and a terrific marriage. They prescribed pain killers and anti-depressants. The side effects of the drugs caused her to feel "spaced out." Something was definitely wrong, but no one had a clue. Who would have ever guessed food allergy?

What you eat *can* make a difference. The proper non-allergenic diet can boost your health, increase your performance, and improve your overall physical appearance. There are a number of documented cases where proper attention to food allergy alleviated a host of physical illnesses, including headaches, asthma, chronic skin conditions, and bowel problems. In other instances, the correct diet brought about emotional well-being, greater energy, and clearer thinking. Even athletes at the peak of physical conditioning have reported a surge of strength upon following a proper diet. The possibilities are unlimited, but if you want to find out whether following a food allergy diet can make *you* feel better, you must motivate *yourself* to do something about it. No one is going to do it for you!

This book will help you to uncover latent food allergy without costing you a fortune in blood or skin tests. With *Hidden Food Allergies* as your guide, you can discover which foods are unhealthy for you and which ones are safe to eat. Discovering foods that may be harmful will no longer be a guessing game.

The following chapters will provide answers to these questions:

•Do I have food allergy?

•To what extent does food allergy contribute to my health problems?

•What specific food(s) should I avoid?

•How can I treat my food allergy?

THE PROBLEM

After dealing with food allergy problems for years, I realized that there are two stumbling blocks. One is a person's not knowing that food allergy may be responsible for his symptoms. Unaware of this possibility, he makes no effort to investigate it. The other is a mistaken belief that poor health is due to food allergy. Such individuals go through life treating themselves for a food allergy that doesn't exist, thus needlessly complicating their lives and delaying the search for what is truly responsible for their poor health.

You may think that discovering whether or not you suffer from a food allergy would be obvious. It isn't. There are many factors that make it complex. There are both immediate and delayed reactions. There are reactions to single foods, multiple foods, and food combinations. At certain times of the year a food can produce symptoms, while at other times it won't. Cooked foods may cause symptoms, whereas natural foods may not. With so many possibilities, it's no wonder that doctors and patients often throw up their hands in frustration.

Because food allergy is so complex, people have turned to various skin and blood tests for an easy answer. Many doctors and patients believe that advanced scientific techniques will answer their questions. For many types of disease science holds the answer, but in Chapter 5 you will learn why skin and blood tests cannot diagnose food allergy correctly. There is no doubt that the skin and blood tests are fast, but they are only 20% accurate. A doctor who is asked to order a test that is accurate only 20% of the time will not know how to interpret the results.

This book will tell you everything you need to know to find and treat hidden food allergy, using nothing more than common sense. This technique can be learned and performed by any person of any age, and it can be completed in just three weeks. Three weeks to learn the answer to a question that can change the way you feel and improve your health for the rest of your life!

In order to feel better you must learn and understand the facts about food allergy, and ignore the fiction. Don't be one of those who suffers needlessly because of misdiagnosis or mis-understanding. Don't be one of those who relies on expensive but inaccurate tests. Although simple, these tests are grossly misleading since they have a high rate of false positive and false negative results. Later on in the book, you will learn the reason why.

If you wish to consult a health care practitioner in addition to using this book, you should be aware that there are five types of allergists. In Chapter 3 you will learn how to choose the one that would be best for you.

THE ONE HUNDRED PERCENT SOLUTION

In the area of food allergy there are two unassailable facts. **One: If you don't know what food you are allergic to, you cannot do anything about it. Two: If you do know what food you are allergic to, it is within your power to improve your health.**

In Chapters 2 through 6 you will find a guaranteed way of telling whether you have food allergy and to what extent your poor health, your disability, or your illness is due to it. You will learn how to carefully select the foods that are most likely causing your food allergy. Then you will learn the proper way to eliminate them from your diet. After this step you will be taught how to judge the degree of improvement. This is crucial in deciding whether food allergy is contributing significantly to your health problem.

If food allergy is a major factor, Chapter 7 will tell you how to pinpoint the specific food that is causing your problem. There is a systematic approach that will enable you to zero in on the culprit. Knowledge is power. Knowledge of the offending food will give you the power to control the way you feel. You will not be at the mercy of forces you don't understand and that are holding you back and dragging you down.

In Chapter 8 you will learn a sensible way to treat your hidden food allergies. There are numerous bizarre and difficult methods of treating food allergy that are available. You will learn how to avoid related foods and how to master your food allergy instead of allowing food allergy to master *you*. Anyone can prescribe a diet of water and celery, but for most people this cure would be intolerable!

At this point patients usually ask if there is a simple way to diagnose and cure food allergy. They want to know why the federal government hasn't spent more money investigating food allergy, why new tests haven't been invented, and where they can go to find a simple answer.

The government doesn't have to spend money, and you don't have to go anywhere. We already have the technical know-how to discover the answers, but since each individual has a different body and a different metabolism, the answer will vary from person to person. You cannot assume that what helped a neighbor, relative, or friend will help you. You cannot assume that what helped your favorite television or movie star, or even your own doctor, will help you. It's a curious fact of human nature, but if a Hollywood star proclaims that he stopped eating wheat and felt better, many fans would probably conclude that they, too, should stop eating wheat products. You must focus on yourself and find the solution to your own problem.

I wrote this book to answer the questions of both doctors and patients. There is a lot of information about food, diet, allergy, nutrition, and health, but keeping up with it all can be a full-time job. It's no wonder that there is so much confusion and misunderstanding!

The correct method for diagnosing food allergy is straightforward. You may not realize it, but each one of you is aware of the rules. With step-by-step guidance from this book you will find the answers you have been searching for. To diagnose your food allergy, all you need is common sense and about three weeks. Doctors are often so busy caring for seriously ill patients that they cannot spend the necessary time to explain the method to their patients. This book will point you in the right direction and lead you to the final diagnosis and treatment.

Many people work backwards. They make the error of searching for a food to which they are allergic *before* knowing whether they even suffer from food allergy! Avoiding specific foods is proper in the treatment phase, but not in the diagnosis phase. This is a guaranteed method to obtain poor results. Beginning the search for hidden food allergy by eliminating one food at a time until the culprit is found can lead to a situation in which a person eliminates one food after another over a period of months, only to discover that he did not have food allergy in the first place. Don't you fall into this trap!

Surveys and medical studies show that over one third of the population has allergies. This makes allergy a widespread illness. It affects people of all ages. It strikes infants, children, teenagers, adults, and seniors. Contrary to popular opinion, it can begin at any time of life. Although it may come as a shock that a person could develop allergy to a food after twenty years of eating it, this is how allergies begin. After continual exposure, allergically-susceptible individuals develop allergy, while non-susceptible people can eat as much as they want for as long as they want and not become allergic. The latter group may become overweight, but they won't become allergic!

Doctors call this exposure and build-up to an allergic state the period of sensitization. After becoming sensitized, the individual is then at risk of experiencing symptoms when he eats the allergenic food. Thus, it is never too early or too late to investigate food allergy.

To give you an idea of the wide variety of symptoms that food allergy can create, a list of them appears below. You might find it hard to believe that foods can cause so many different problems, but in every case it has proven to be true.

"YOU'VE GOT TO BE KIDDING!"

When people read this list, they are skeptical. Because the list is so all-inclusive, you would think that allergists are the only type of physician a person would ever need! It should come as no surprise, however, that foods can cause so much trouble. Considering the amount of foods, chemicals, and preservatives that are poured into our systems each day, it is a miracle that anyone could escape life *without* a food allergy.

There are many that do escape allergy. In fact, less than half the population has food allergy. But statistics are meaningless when it comes to an individual. If you are one out of the three that has food allergy, it is 100% for you. Therefore, each person should consider whether he has food allergy without regard to statistics that try to minimize the problem by stating that you have only a 33% chance of being allergic. You should adopt a self-centered attitude. No matter what the odds and what the experts say, tell yourself that you want to achieve the best health you can. Part of your program will be a commitment to investigate food allergy and follow the path that bona fide experiments have shown will uncover food allergy. If the path proves that you have food allergy, then you will accept the results and do your best to discover the offending foods. If the path proves that you do not have significant food allergy, then you will accept this result, too. At the end of your investigation there will be no doubt one way or the other.

As you read the following list, you must remember that other illnesses can cause or contribute to many of the same problems that appear here. It is a common mistake to separate the question "Do I have food allergy?" from the question "To what extent does food allergy contribute to my problem?"

If you are experiencing a symptom on the list, food allergy may be responsible for 10% of that symptom and another illness responsible for 90%. In this case you would not want to spend 90% of your time, money, and effort searching for a food that will yield only 10% relief. You would first want to work on what would relieve 90% of the problem. On the other hand, if food allergy is 90% of your problem, then it would be worth the effort to find out what food is making you feel so ill.

The following list is not a quiz. If you have one or several symptoms, then you are a candidate for food allergy, and it would be worth your while to find out more about it. Some of these symptoms are commonly due to food allergy, and some are not.

It takes three weeks to discover the answer, and it can be done by yourself, in your home, without completely disrupting your life or draining your pocketbook.

As you read the list, ask yourself if you are aware of any symptoms that may be missing. I obtained this information from my own experience and from published reports, but I would be the first to admit that I have not seen or read everything. There are undoubtedly rare problems that have not come to my attention. At the end of the list are some blank lines. Write down any symptoms that you think might be due to food allergy.

Signs and Symptoms That Can Indicate Hidden Food Allergy

Head:
____ Headaches
____ Sinusitis
____ Faintness
____ Dizziness
____ A feeling of fullness in the head
____ Excessive drowsiness
____ Insomnia

Eyes:
____ Itchy eyes
____ Watery eyes
____ Blurred vision
____ Baggy, swollen eyelids

Ears:
____ Ringing in ears
____ Earache
____ Fullness of ears
____ Fluid in middle ear
____ Loss of hearing
____ Recurring ear infections
____ Itching
____ Drainage from ear

Nose:
____ Runny nose
____ Stuffy nose
____ Excessive mucus
____ Postnasal drainage

Throat:
____ Sore throat
____ Hoarseness
____ Chronic cough
____ Gagging
____ Clearing of throat
____ Ticklish feeling in throat

Mouth:
____ Canker sores
____ Itching of roof of mouth
____ Bleeding gums
____ Mouth sores

Neck:
____ Swollen glands

Heart:
____ Palpitations
____ Increased heart rate
____ Irregular heartbeat

Lungs:
_____ Asthma
_____ Congestion in chest
_____ Wheezing and whistling
sounds in the lungs
_____ Difficulty breathing
_____ Coughing

Gastrointestinal:
_____ Nausea
_____ Vomiting
_____ Diarrhea
_____ Constipation
_____ Bloating
_____ Belching
_____ Colitis
_____ Flatulence (passing
of gas)
_____ Feeling of fullness
_____ Abdominal pains

Urinary Tract:
_____ Pain during urination
_____ Burning
_____ Infections
_____ Frequency of urination
_____ Urgency of urination

Reproductive Organs:
_____ Vaginal itching
_____ Vaginal discharge
_____ Menstrual problems

Skin:
_____ Hives
_____ Rashes
_____ Eczema
_____ Dermatitis
_____ Acne
_____ Dandruff
_____ Loss of hair

_____ Dark circles under
the eyes

Other Symptoms:
_____ Chronic fatigue
_____ Lethargy
_____ Weakness
_____ Muscle aches and pains
_____ Arthritis
_____ Swelling of hands, feet,
or ankles
_____ Motion sickness

Weight:
_____ Difficulty losing weight
_____ Difficulty gaining weight
_____ Fluid retention
_____ Hunger
_____ Binge eating
_____ Being overweight
_____ Being underweight

Psychological:
_____ Anxiety
_____ Panic attacks
_____ Depression
_____ Crying jags
_____ Aggressive behavior
_____ Irritability
_____ Mental dullness
_____ Mental lethargy
_____ Confusion
_____ Excessive daydreaming
_____ Hyperactivity
_____ Restlessness
_____ Learning disabilities
_____ Poor work habits
_____ Slurred speech
_____ Stuttering
_____ Inability to concentrate

____ Indifference
____ Stress

Learning:
____ Underachievement
____ Inability to concentrate
____ Disorganization
____ Easily distractable
____ Inability to follow
directions
____ Short attention span
____ Illogical thought
processes
____ Dyslexia
____ Slow, disorganized
speech
____ No awareness of cause-
effect
____ Perceptual problems

Characteristics:
____ Excitable
____ Impulsive
____ Reckless
____ Disruptive

Aggressive:
____ Unreasonable
____ Argumentative

____ Uncooperative
____ No self-control
____ Bad temper
____ Cries easily
____ Talks incessantly
____ Interrupts
____ Bed wets
____ Poor sleep habits
____ Easily frustrated
____ Jekyll-Hyde personality

Motor:
____ High energy level
____ Touches constantly
____ Clumsy
____ Uncoordinated
____ Fidgety
____ Crib rocks
____ Head rocks
____ Eye-hand coordination
problems

Other:
_____
_____
_____
_____
_____

2

Suspecting
Food Allergy

*Johnny's teachers couldn't control him. He walked around when
he was supposed to be sitting. He talked when he was supposed
to be silent. He didn't pay attention. At home he was constantly
in motion. The doctor prescribed medication for an indefinite
period of time, until a school counselor suggested that food allergy
could be the problem. It was.*

If any of the symptoms listed in the previous chapter sound
familiar, then you should consider the possibility that you may
have hidden food allergy. Anyone who suspects food allergy
must consider two types of reactions: immediate-type food allergy and delayed-type food allergy.

IMMEDIATE-TYPE FOOD ALLERGY

In the immediate-type reaction, the individual experiences
symptoms within seconds after eating the offending food. Every
time he eats the food, the reaction occurs. Some well-known
examples are hives that appear after eating shellfish, itching of
the mouth that comes from fresh fruit, or vomiting that occurs
from eating peanuts. These reactions usually subside within an
hour. They are easy to pinpoint because the reaction occurs so
soon and so consistently after ingestion that a cause-and-effect

relationship is usually apparent to everyone.

People who suffer from immediate-type food reactions do not have to be convinced that food can cause such reactions. They know it!

DELAYED-TYPE FOOD ALLERGY

Delayed-type reactions occur hours or even days after a food is ingested. In certain cases, several kinds of foods must be ingested in combination in order to provoke the reaction. For this type of reaction, it is almost impossible to see a cause-and-effect relationship. It's difficult enough to remember what you ate several days ago, not to mention which of the many foods might have triggered your symptoms. The time lapse between eating a food and experiencing symptoms naturally causes people to doubt that food could be responsible for their problems. Until I learned more about it, I thought it was strange myself!

When we eat a food, the body breaks it down into many small particles and eventually into chemicals like sugar, amino acids, and fats so that the body cells can utilize the substances. Thus, the body changes each food we eat into dozens of different byproducts.

These chemicals and byproducts can be allergenic. It is the time lapse between eating the food and the body's creation of these products that accounts for the delay in the reaction. The body of the allergy-prone individual must wait until the allergenic byproduct is created from the ingested food. You will see later how this fact explains why skin and blood tests (which are very reliable for diagnosing allergy to airborne materials such as pollens, dust, animal dander, and molds) are so unreliable for diagnosing food allergy.

ARE DOCTORS SKEPTICAL?

When I was in medical school, I learned a lot about immediate-type reactions but nothing about the possibility of delayed-type reactions. As a result, I didn't consider them. Only after I studied allergy did I realize how common it is for foods to provoke symptoms days later.

Traditional medical school training provides scant instruction in nutrition. Courses concentrate on the pathology of diseases, diagnosis of illness, proper use of medication, and correct surgical techniques. The idea of teaching preventive health through diets and exercise has been a low priority. Medical schools are becoming aware of this deficiency, and many of them are now changing their curriculums.

At the present time, however, numerous physicians are unfamiliar with the relationship among diet, disease, and food allergy. Although this is largely the fault of the system, the one who suffers is the patient whose food allergies are being ignored. Many patients have been through the experience of a complete examination and, when no life-threatening disease is found, are reassured that the tests turned out normal and that there is nothing to worry about. Such an individual may assume that he's got a psychological problem, since his physical examination, blood tests, and x-rays came out fine. Although a person may not have a psychological problem to begin with, he can develop one as a result of wondering how it is possible to have a clean bill of health and yet feel so miserable.

Such patients are often pushed aside because unraveling their problems can be complex and time-consuming. It's not because the doctors don't care. They care deeply, and feel badly when they cannot do more. But they are victims of minimal training in allergy and nutrition, too many demands, and too little time.

If food problems were short-lived, perhaps it would not be so important to diagnose them. When a person has insomnia or gastrointestinal symptoms a few days out of the year, it isn't worth a lot of time and money trying to find a solution. When the illness is persistent and debilitating, however, you cannot afford to ignore it because it can take over your life. Time that should be spent enjoying yourself is instead devoted to an exhausting battle to maintain good health. It's especially frustrating if you must do it by yourself.

Not all doctors ignore food allergy. Many are astute and recognize that their patients are suffering from food allergy. In such cases they often recommend that their patients keep a daily diary of the foods they eat and any reactions that occur.

This type of investigation is suitable when the food allergy is of the immediate-type. On the other hand, immediate-type reactions occur so soon after the person eats the food that the reaction is usually obvious without a diary.

A diary does not help in diagnosing delayed-type reactions. It does not take into account food combinations or the fact that reactions can be delayed several hours or days.

In some situations, a doctor who is aware that there is a food allergy problem may not tell his patient of his suspicion. Reassured by the physical examination and the battery of tests, the doctor may instead tell his patient not to worry. From the perspective of dealing with patients with serious diseases, such advice may be understandable. The doctor's obligation, however, should not end once he has proven that his patient does not have an acute or potentially deadly disease. His next question should be, "If I don't have the time or training to take care of this person's allergy problem, where should I send him?"

Don't jump to the conclusion that food allergy is at the root of *every* unexplained illness. A person doesn't have to be a medical school graduate to know that different diseases can produce identical symptoms. For example, headaches can be due to a brain tumor, stress, a sinus infection, or eye strain. When the worst possibility, such as a brain tumor, is ruled out, you or your doctor should continue down the list until you reach the correct diagnosis.

This is where *you*, the patient, must often take part in your own care. Sometimes doctors will stop short on the list. If you experience problems or symptoms that no one has explained to your satisfaction, then you must consider that perhaps hidden food allergy is contributing to your poor health.

YOU MAY BE AT FAULT!

Patients, as well as doctors, can be at fault in ignoring food allergy. Some are convinced that they have it, but make no effort to prove it. Some don't know and don't care. Some have it, but don't believe it.

A person can mistakenly believe that he has food allergy when he reads or hears of an individual whose symptoms are similar to his and has a food allergy. On the "misery loves company" theory, he might conclude that he, too, suffers from the same problem. Without attempting to double-check, he may restrict his diet needlessly and sometimes harmfully. One young woman, whom I was asked to consult, had been told that her long-standing clinical depression was due to food allergy. After careful analysis using the plan outlined in this book, it became clear that foods were not her problem. She had wasted four years trying to modify her diet when she should have been in psychological therapy or on medication.

In other cases, patients don't hear about the kinds of problems that food allergy can cause, so they miss the opportunity to improve their health. There was a family whose child had uncontrolled hyperactivity for many years, until an alert teacher mentioned that food allergy could be a contributing factor to behavioral problems. Once the offending foods were eliminated, there was immediate improvement (to the great relief of the family, the school, and the child himself).

Still others know they have food allergy but refuse to do anything about it, similar to the stubborn smokers and drinkers who are intellectually aware of the danger but refuse to change their bad habits.

FACE UP TO THE PROBLEM

There is no excuse for ignoring food allergy. Neither doctors nor patients should claim that this possibility did not cross their minds or that it would be too time-consuming or costly to figure out. The most important step in finding food allergies is to be aware that food allergy *can* be causing your symptoms. This should be easy because the list of symptoms and diseases that have been attributed to food allergy includes anything that affects the body from head to toe.

No matter how far-fetched it may seem, you can suspect a food allergy when you have virtually any abnormal health condition. This does not necessarily mean that food allergy is responsible for your condition—only that you should suspect it.

You should not apologize for being suspicious and wanting to investigate this possibility. Many individuals believe that unless they have a dreadful disease they are not entitled to look into food allergy.

Maybe I shouldn't be bothering the doctor.

Maybe I'm overreacting.

Maybe I'm not that bad.

If you have been suffering with a problem and have been left on your own to cope with it, you have nothing to lose and a lot to gain by learning whether food allergy is at the bottom of it. Food allergies go undiagnosed because people are ignorant of the possibility, are too embarrassed to mention such a bizarre idea, or are ridiculed by relatives, neighbors, and friends for believing that supposedly healthy foods can be making them ill.

You must overcome ignorance, embarrassment, and denial and allow yourself to suspect that food allergy *can* be the cause of your problem. Once you can stick up for yourself, you are ready to begin the search for hidden food allergy.

3
Writing Down the Symptoms

Brian, a type-A executive of a large company, had periodic episodes of dizziness. He heard about hidden food allergy and decided to investigate. Impatient and anxious to begin, he decided to do the diet without determining first how frequently the dizziness occurred. As usual, he threw every ounce of energy into the diet. At the end he thought he was a lot better, but on some days the dizziness (although it seemed milder) was still present. Brian could have kicked himself for being too eager to start the diet and unwilling to spend the ten minutes it took to write down his baseline symptoms so that he could judge his degree of improvement. Brian had wasted three weeks of his time.

Your first task in the hunt for hidden food allergy is to write down your symptoms. This might seem like an unnecessary step, but you will not know whether your search has been successful unless you know what you are trying to achieve. When you put a jigsaw puzzle together, you know you have been successful when your finished puzzle matches the picture on the box cover.

It's the same way with food allergy. You must figure out what health problem you are hoping to improve. If you wanted to run a faster mile, you would write down your current speed for comparison. If you wanted to sleep better, you would write down your current sleep pattern. If you wanted to stop diarrhea, you would write down your present bowel habits. If you wanted to breathe easier from asthma, you would write down your present problem. This is the point at which you must decide which symptoms or group of symptoms you wish to alleviate.

Begin by writing down the symptoms that bother you the most. You would not go on a trip without first knowing your destination, and you cannot start a search for hidden food allergy unless you know what you hope to accomplish. In both cases you would not know whether you had arrived where you wanted to be.

Think about it for a moment. How will you know you've reached your goal if you don't know what your goal is?

What is bothering you? Your goal is to eradicate certain health problems. You, alone, know how you feel, and now you must analyze your situation. You must write down the symptoms that bother you, starting with the most bothersome and ending with the least bothersome. Also write down how often the symptoms occur. Once you have done this, you will be able to judge when your symptoms have changed.

Food Allergy Baseline

Ranking	Symptom Description	Frequency of Symptoms Before Doing Diet (days/week)	Symptom-Free Interval Before Doing Diet

The chart on pages 18 and 19 will help you to do this. It is called the Food Allergy Baseline (FAB) because it is a FABulous way to begin the hunt for your food allergy. The FAB points you in the right direction and tells you when you have arrived at your destination.

THE FOOD ALLERGY BASELINE (FAB)

If you need help figuring out how to write down your symptoms, return to the list of symptoms in Chapter 1. Read through the list and enter the ones that apply in Column 2 (Column 2 is the one labelled "Symptom Description").

If you have a symptom that was inadvertently left out of this book, be sure to include it. Be specific. Do not write "stomach trouble." Ask yourself if you experience pain, burning, nausea, or gas. Write down each description that applies. If you have two types of headaches, enter them separately (e.g. "left-sided pounding" and "top of the head steady"). If you have arthritis, write "left elbow pain," "right knee swollen," "fingers stiff," etc. Use extra paper if necessary.

Food Allergy Baseline (Continued)

Frequency of Symptoms After Doing Diet (days/week)	Percent Improvement on Third Week of Diet	Could Have Improved On Its Own	No Chance It Improved On Its Own

At this point you will only fill out Columns 1 through 4. You will return to Columns 5 through 8 later, so put a paper clip on the first page of the FAB to enable you to find it easily.

Next go to Column 3. Write down the number of days per week that the symptom occurs. This will vary from week to week and month to month, so consider the previous four weeks and determine the average. For example:

> sneezing   4 days out of 7 = 4/7
> pounding headache   1 day out of 7 = 1/7
> steady headache   3 days out of 7 = 3/7

If your symptom occurs infrequently, write the average. For example:

> fatigue   2 days a month = 2/30
> hives   4 days a month = 4/30

In Column 1 put an asterisk or use a colored pencil to mark which symptoms are the most uncomfortable. Think of it this way. For which problem would you give $100 to anyone who could relieve you of it? Which ones are worth only $15 because they don't bother you that much? If you want you can rank them 1, 2, 3, 4, 5, 6, 7, 8, 9, 10—1 being the worst and 10 the mildest. Or you can have three rated 1 and the rest rated 10.

Finally, in Column 4 write down your best estimate of how long you can go without that symptom. Can you go one day, one week, one month, or longer? This column may seem insignificant, but it is extraordinarily important in determining whether you improved while you were following the diet. Think carefully about your answer.

Ignore Columns 5 through 8 for now. This is your Food Allergy Baseline, and you will use these facts to determine whether you have hidden food allergy.

Helpful Hint #1   Ranking Your Symptoms

It is especially important that you think carefully about how you rank your symptoms in Column 1 from the most bothersome to the least bothersome. If you have not done this carefully, you will commit one of the most common errors that occurs in diagnosing food allergy, and you will be off to a bad start.

Frequently, when patients seek advice from their doctors, the doctor is so busy that he cannot take the time to carefully rank each patient's problem. When faced with a variety of symptoms, the doctor may prescribe something for the one that is easiest to treat. Assuming that this symptom is the most bothersome one, the patient will obtain satisfactory relief. But if the doctor happens to focus on a minor symptom, the patient would achieve only partial relief.

A favorite example of mine is the middle-aged man I saw who had been treated with immunizing injections for tree pollen. As expected, the injections stopped his sneezing, but his headaches—which were the primary reason he had come for treatment—continued full-force. The health care provider had made the mistake of assuming that allergy to trees was responsible for both the sneezing *and* the headaches. As it turned out, hidden food allergy was causing the headaches and the injections were unnecessary. The diagnosis was completely wrong. A devil's advocate could argue that the springtime sneezing had been cured, but it would not change the fact that the man's year-round incapacitating headaches continued out of control. When I questioned the patient about this, he admitted that he would have gladly put up with two weeks of sneezing if he could rid himself of the headaches that were occurring every day of his life.

Another patient had bowel problems and itchy eyes. Upon allergy testing she had been found to be allergic to weeds, so her doctor began a series of weed injections. But her doctor neglected the basics and missed the fact that the itchy eyes were a minor nuisance in the spring while her year-round bowel problem was due to food allergy.

Finding a patient whose treatment has been misdirected is not uncommon. It's easy for both a doctor and a patient to become sidetracked because multiple problems are often present and it's hard to sort them out in a busy medical practice.

I have found in my own practice that I must often ask the same question several different ways to be sure I understand what the major problem is, how frequently it is happening, and how significant it is.

Take your time as you rank your symptoms. Remember, this will tell you when you have reached your goal.

Helpful Hint #2   Choosing an Allergist

If you would like additional help and wish to consult an allergist, you may do so. Many patients prefer to have a doctor help them with their allergy. Some read this book and then seek advice. Others see their doctor, who then recommends this book.

In the United States there are five categories of health care professionals who provide allergy advice. In order to help you choose the type that is best suited for you, I have categorized them based on the extent of their training in caring for allergic diseases. Of all the health care providers in the United States, only 3,000 have been trained for allergy treatment. So the chances are better than 80% that you will obtain allergy care from someone who has not been properly trained.

Many people are embarrassed to ask what kind of training their doctor has had, frightened to question whether he is the right person to handle their particular problem, or nervous about what he will think if they ask for a second opinion. People who wouldn't hesitate to ask their auto mechanic such questions are afraid to ask when it comes to their own bodies. Instead, they permit an untrained allergy provider to prescribe their treatment. If the treatment is successful, there is no harm done. For example, if a bartender told a customer that he should avoid peanuts after the customer had just broken out in hives after eating a handful, the advice would be sound. The customer would not have to undergo great expense in order to take care of his allergy. Unfortunately, much of the advice from untrained people is incorrect.

Beware of phonies! Because allergy seems like such a simple concept on the surface, it's no wonder that many health care providers want to get into the act. Many of them mistakenly believe that allergy treatment means doing a few tests, ordering an allergy serum, and letting their nurses give allergy shots. In the United States there is an increasing number of physicians who call themselves allergists but who, in fact, lack proper training. By being too busy or too uninterested to keep up with the latest advances, such health care providers waste the millions of dollars and thousands of man-hours that have been spent over the past two decades in understanding and improving allergy care.

There are two types of certified allergists, Type I and Type II. Both have passed an examination in allergy and are officially Board Certified in Allergy and Immunology, but Type I has had two additional years of supervised training in one of fifty special University programs in the United States or Canada. Type II has not. The two years of allergy training comes *after* the doctor has had the three to four years of training required to become a Board Certified Internist, Pediatrician, or Family Practitioner.

You might wonder how a physician could be officially Board Certified and be untrained. In the early 1970's, when the Internal Medicine Allergy Board and the Pediatric Allergy Board agreed to merge, there were many physicians who were practicing allergy but were not considered eligible to take the qualifying examination because in many cases they did not even have the three or four years of training that are required for Board Certification in Internal Medicine, Pediatrics, or Family Practice. They sued the Board for restraint of trade and won their case in court. Despite these physicians' lack of training, the Board was ordered to allow them to take the examination under a so-called grandfather provision. Many physicians attended cram courses, passed the exam, and thus became Board Certified Allergists. (If you want to learn whether a person who claims to be a Board Certified Allergist has had the extra two years of training, you may write to the American Board of Allergy and Immunology, University City Science Center, 3624 Market St., Philadelphia, PA 19104.) See Appendix E for some other useful addresses.

Remember that many of the untrained physicians can be helpful. Seeing a doctor who has had the extra two years of training may not be necessary in your case. Nevertheless, you are entitled to a full disclosure of your doctor's background and training so you can make an informed decision. Remember: You are entrusting your health to his care.

Type III allergists are health care providers such as family practitioners; ear, nose, and throat surgeons; internists; chiropractors; and acupuncturists. These professionals must learn a little about everything. There are many half-day to two-day allergy seminars where they can learn how to help you or assist you in deciding whether you ought to see a specialist.

It's not easy to decide when your problem can be handled by your family practitioner, pediatrician, or chiropractor and when you must see one of the Type I or Type II allergists. That is a decision *you* must make. You are the patient with the problem. You must decide what is in your best interest.

If you are one of the many people who is afraid of hurting your doctor's feelings by asking for a referral or who assumes that your doctor would initiate one if he wanted you to be seen, you must overcome these ideas. I have never met a doctor who became angry at his patient because the patient asked to see a specialist. Often, doctors wait for the patient to ask on the assumption that if the symptoms were that bothersome the patient would request a referral. It reminds me of two people about to enter an elevator, each one waiting for the other to go first. Meanwhile, the doors close and neither one gets on.

Type IV allergists call themselves clinical ecologists or environmental allergists. Other ecologists must train them because universities in the United States do not offer this type of instruction. The typical tests (cytotoxic, sublingual, and certain muscle tests) and typical treatment (injections of chemicals, neutralizing shots, and sublingual drops) that ecologists prescribe have been proven unreliable in the vast majority of cases. Once in a while a patient will claim that he has benefited from ecology treatments. However, controlled studies do not support such claims. It is extremely rare to find a person who truly has these kinds of allergies.

There are many individuals who react to chemicals in the air, but the reactions are not allergic reactions. They are toxic and irritant reactions from excessive levels of fumes, vapors, gases, and particles, and should not be confused with allergy.

Type V allergists consist of neighbors, friends, relatives, and pharmacists. Allergy is such a common problem that everyone seems to have an opinion on it. Sometimes their opinions are correct, and sometimes they're not. You can judge by the results. If your bartender's advice to stop eating peanuts solves your problem, then no further care is necessary. But if your problem is not solved, you should seek qualified help.

Don't Get Overcharged!

Interestingly, the cost of an allergy examination and subsequent treatment is frequently inversely related to the quality and thoroughness of the doctor's training. Type IV ecologists often do expensive testing by cytotoxic, neutralizing technique, sublingual drops, or total environmental isolation. The cost can be anywhere from $2,000 to $10,000. In contrast, a Type I allergist usually charges $350 to $475 for a complete exam. The Type II and Type III allergists are in-between.

It seems contradictory that the doctors with less training charge more money, but they rely on highly expensive and inaccurate testing instead of the patient's history, the physical exam, experience, and common sense. For food allergy, the different skin, blood, sublingual drop, muscle, and neutralizing dose tests are inaccurate. They aren't dangerous, but they don't tell us what we want to know.

Patients often forget that it isn't the test that's important—it's the *interpretation* of the test. A blood pressure of 60/40 might be normal in a small child lying in bed, while in an adult it would indicate cardiovascular shock. A hemoglobin of 18 might be normal in an individual residing on a mountain where the air is thin, but would indicate a blood disease in someone living at sea level.

In an era of such sophistication, patients expect to have the latest tests done. They may not, however, be in a position to judge the usefulness of those tests. Doctors are subject to advertising and promotion, and unless they read the literature and experiments carefully, they can fall into the same trap as patients who rely on newspaper stories, magazine articles, and advertising that promote the "newest" test methods. Many physicians are pressured into ordering these tests without asking whether they are of any use. They may be unaware of the high frequency of false positive and false negative results when such food tests are performed. They may make the mistake of assuming that a positive test always indicates a cause-and-effect relationship, although careful studies have repeatedly proven that the three blood tests, the four skin tests, the sublingual tests, and the neutralizing dose tests for food allergy are no guarantee that food allergy is present.

Moreover, these tests cost money. In the United States we are so used to throwing money at a problem that we sometimes forget that money and new technology do not necessarily get results. And, in the case of food allergy, money and high-tech tests are *not* the answer.

There is no simple way for a patient to avoid falling into the hands of a health care provider who orders costly food allergy tests without fully understanding the implications and drawbacks of such tests. A professional degree on a letterhead or on an office wall is no guarantee that this individual has had the time to attend scientific meetings, where he can keep up with the literature. A degree does not, as you have already learned, necessarily mean the professional has had proper training. How often have doctors tried new treatments or drugs, only to find that they did not live up to their expectations?

I know of some trained Type I allergists who were swayed by the seductive advertising of companies that promote blood test methods for diagnosing food allergy. If the Type I allergist can be convinced by high pressure ads, think how easy it would be to convince the other types!

Choosing an allergist is the same as choosing someone to service your car, your television, or your taxes. You can go to someone who has taught himself, someone who has had minimal training, or someone who is fully trained. You can always get lucky with regard to the practitioner you choose, but you'll be better off if you consult someone who has been properly trained.

Forget high-tech. Forget shortcuts that don't work. With your Food Allergy Baseline in hand, you're ready to get down to business.

4

Selecting a Test Diet

Margaret couldn't motivate herself to begin her test diet until she knew what food bothered her. However, she couldn't identify the offending food until she started her diet. She had boxed herself into a classic vicious circle. She kept thinking up excuses to avoid beginning an elimination diet, and suffered as she did so.

Once you have written down your symptoms, you must find out whether they're being caused by food allergy. To do so, you must eliminate certain foods from your body. This chapter tells you how to decide what foods you should avoid. There are two ways of doing this. You can eliminate many foods at a time, or you can eliminate each food separately.

The vast majority of health care practitioners recommend eliminating each food separately in order to pinpoint the specific food affecting their patient. But *you* should not begin this way. You mustn't fall into the trap of being so anxious to discover the specific food that is bothering you that you don't stop long enough to consider that you may not even have food allergy in the first place! It's like bringing your automobile in for repair and telling the mechanic to replace the engine without first finding out if you need a new one.

The first step in the successful diagnosis and treatment of food allergy is proving that food allergy is the cause of the

disease. This commonsense rule is commonly ignored. Both patients and physicians can make the unpardonable error of assuming that food allergy is present without proving it. Such guessing inevitably leads to improper treatment and, even worse, can lead to the neglect of another illness that may be the true cause of your condition. You cannot avoid a food and thereby hope to alleviate an illness that is not caused by a food allergy. (For example, if you had diabetes, you could stop eating hundreds of foods, but would not alter your diabetic condition.) My important advice to you is *not to be in a rush to discover the offending food*.

There are two basic principles that should be understood as you investigate the possibility of food allergies.

Eliminating a food. This first principle has withstood the test of time. When you avoid a substance to which you are allergic, the substance cannot affect you. No one has ever disproven this rule. No matter how allergic you might be to peanuts, nothing will happen to you as long as you don't eat them. By the same logic, if you have eliminated a certain food from your diet and do not feel better, then the food cannot be responsible for your symptoms.

Eliminating a lot of foods. This second principle is less familiar, for it seems to defy all logic. The usual method of doing an elimination diet is to eliminate one food at a time. Otherwise, it is impossible to figure out which food is the culprit.

Consider the following facts, though.

What if a person reacts to combinations of foods? In such a case, he will never discover that he has hidden food allergy. Eliminating one food at a time will lead him to the false conclusion that he is not allergic to food, when in fact he is.

What if a person is not allergic to foods? In this case he will go through many tests, many doctor's visits, many months, and many dollars looking for something that isn't there.

Although this second principle sounds unreasonable and backward, it saves much time, money, and effort. If you do have food allergy, you'll find out for sure. If you don't have food allergy, you'll find out sooner rather than later.

What if you eliminate a food for only one or two days instead of the full three weeks? In this case you will not detect delayed food allergy reactions. The body takes time to process foods.

There can be a delay between the ingestion of a food and the resulting reaction. If this diet is not maintained for three weeks, you might miss a delayed reaction.

Equally important is the healing factor. When the body reacts to a food, certain changes take place. Once the noxious stimulus is removed, it can take time for the body to heal enough so that you can recognize a cause-and-effect relationship. Take the example of an acne lesion on the skin that is due to food. Although no new lesions may occur within a few days of discontinuing the allergenic food, it can take a week or longer for the old acne lesions to heal enough to detect an improvement.

No matter what is said, some patients won't give up their burning desire to undergo a lot of expensive, inaccurate tests before they know whether food allergy is their problem. Even if the blood and skin tests *are* ordered, a person should do the diet test anyway. No one should rely on results that are 20% accurate when there is a test that is 100% accurate! Don't be conned into doing blood, skin, neutralizing dose, sublingual drops, or muscle tests for food allergies.

NO EXCUSES, PLEASE!

The diet you must follow is called the General Elimination Diet. It eliminates several groups of foods simultaneously, and remember—its sole purpose is to learn whether you have food allergy, *not* to pinpoint a particular allergenic food.

The more traditional type of diet you will encounter elsewhere is the Specific Elimination Diet, which eliminates a single food. Remember—its purpose is to learn what food is causing problems. The Specific Elimination Diet is the one to do *after* you have proven that food allergy is responsible for your problem. You will find that most health care providers begin with the Specific Elimination Diet partly because they don't know any better, partly because their patients expect them to, and partly because they hope to find the offending food. You can see how shortsighted this approach can be. Those people who don't have food allergy would be wasting their time, as well as running the risk of missing food allergy, since eliminating a single food doesn't take into account the well-known fact that food allergies can be multiple and cumulative.

When I tell a patient that he must create a General Elimination Diet and follow it for three weeks, the word "elimination" triggers some of the strangest excuses. I've probably heard them all.

•"It's too hard."

•"It's too impractical."

•"It takes too long."

•"I'll lose too much weight."

•"I'll gain too much weight."

•"I've done diets before."

•"I'm already on a diet."

•"I can't eat these things."

•"I can't avoid these things."

•"I travel too much."

•"I stay at home too much."

•"My family won't put up with it."

•"I can't control what he eats at school."

•"What if my allergies change?"

In the space below, feel free to write down any objections that I seem to have missed. Send me a postcard (in care of the publisher) so I can include your ideas in the next edition!

Now consider all you can gain by doing the diet. Everything has its advantages and disadvantages, and to be fair to yourself you should weigh both sides. You read about the disadvantages that I've heard and wrote down the disadvantages that you perceive. Now do yourself a favor and read the advantages.

ADVANTAGES OF A GENERAL ELIMINATION DIET

If you have a chronic problem and have become fed up with it because it is interfering with your life, your relationships with other people, and how you perform at work and at play, you now have an opportunity to learn—in three weeks—whether hidden food allergy is responsible for your illness. Many individuals have explored all kinds of treatments and have had many different tests that are consistently "normal." Often, they have a medicine closet full of drugs that give no relief and typically produce unpleasant side effects. They have tried vitamins and minerals to no avail. It doesn't make sense to give up a golden opportunity to find out if hidden food allergy is the culprit.

Here is an opportunity to feel better at practically no cost to you. It is simply a commitment of three weeks of your time, and the payoff could mean feeling better for the rest of your life. Not a bad return on a three-week investment!

SELECTING A GENERAL ELIMINATION DIET

In most cases there are two or three groups of foods that are eliminated in a General Elimination Diet. The most common groups are dairy products, chocolate, wheat, corn, and salicylate additives.

Unlike the well-known allergenic foods such as nuts, eggs, citrus, strawberries, and shellfish, which cause immediate-type reactions, the foods listed above more commonly provoke delayed-type reactions—the kind of allergy that is the subject of this book.

There are several reasons for the delay in the reaction. The one that has already been described is the fact that the body must metabolize (or break down) the food into its allergenic form. Another reason for the delay is that, in many cases, it takes an accumulation of food to provoke the symptoms. For example, a highly sensitive person might react to one slice of cheese, while a less sensitive person might require six slices of cheese. In certain cases the allergy sufferer might have to eat two slices a day for three days in a row, as each dose of cheese pecks at the body's defenses until the body succumbs.

Your selection of groups of foods to avoid will change a little bit depending on your age and the type of problem you have, but the correct selection of groups is not as complicated as you might imagine. At this point your goal is to *learn whether or not* you suffer from food allergy and *to what extent*. This is quite different from someone who has already proven he has significant food allergy and wants to pinpoint the offending food.

One reason for hesitation might be, "Could I be allergic to a food not on the list, like celery or tomatoes or wine?" Good question. If a doctor searched the medical literature carefully, he would find a case for anything. Technically, his response would have to be "yes."

If you have any reason to suspect a food that is not in one of the five groups mentioned, add it to the list. Instead of being in doubt, you might as well learn the truth. If you have a friend who is allergic to granola bars, you may avoid granola bars to satisfy your own curiosity. It isn't logical, however, to assume that your body will have the identical allergies as your friend or relative.

Other people claim that they prefer to use superstition to pinpoint the foods that must be eliminated. Patients have often heard that a person craves the food to which he is allergic and therefore eats more of it in a kind of unconscious, masochistic ritual. The idea behind this is that food allergy is similar to narcotic addiction, and the body sends messages to the brain to eat as much of the food as can be tolerated in order to satisfy the addiction. Another superstition is that the body instinctively avoids foods that cause allergy in a kind of natural self-defense. A third possibility is that the body doesn't crave or avoid the food, in which case the person would have no clue as to his hidden food allergy.

All three theories are correct. In some cases people crave the allergenic food, in some they avoid it, and in some they don't know. The dilemma is that doctors do not have a test to tell which body is following what theory. It's as likely to be one as the other, and it is no use to try to figure it out beforehand. After a doctor learns what food caused the food allergy, he can look back and say which patient craved, which patient avoided, and which did not know. The interesting fact is that some patients are combinations. They crave certain foods to which they are ultimately shown to be allergic, and avoid other foods to which they are ultimately shown to be allergic.

You must start with the basics. You must clean out your system of allergenic foods and determine once and for all the degree to which you have food allergy.

There are two General Elimination Diets from which to choose. Adults must avoid all traces of dairy products, chocolate, and salicylate additives (all kinds of chemicals). Children with respiratory problems must avoid all of the above, plus corn products.

If there is a food that you already know affects you with an immediate or delayed reaction, avoid it. If there is a food about which you are curious, avoid it.

In some cases wheat is a problem. Wheat avoidance is described in Appendix A. Some clues that would lead you to avoid wheat are gastrointestinal problems, curiosity about wheat products, or any hint from eating wheat in the past that it may provoke discomfort.

When following a General Elimination Diet, you may choose the method that is easiest for you. There are three possibilities. You can learn what foods are forbidden and avoid them in your diet. Your second choice is to learn what you can eat and not deviate from those foods. Your third choice is to follow a menu plan that tells you which specific meals may be eaten for breakfast, lunch, and dinner.

Appendix A contains complete instructions for the major groups of allergenic foods—dairy, chocolate, corn, wheat, and salicylate additives.

Each diet has been devised as a way of detecting food allergy. These are *test diets*, not treatments. It is extremely important, therefore, that there be *no* violations; otherwise, you cannot determine the role of food allergy in causing your symptoms.

Read labels. Traces of substances can occur in a wide variety of foods. The diets should eliminate every trace of these foods. Although such complete elimination makes the diet more difficult to follow, this phase is a brief test period in order to confirm the diagnosis. Later on you will learn that adequate relief can sometimes be obtained even if you eat trace amounts of allergenic foods *if no other exceptions are made.*

Although these foods are important to the average diet, they can be harmful to a person who is allergic to them. If the diet works and the foods continue to be eliminated, you may need to obtain supplements, but it is not necessary at this point.

Dairy-Chocolate-Salicylate Additive Diet

For the dairy-chocolate-salicylate additive diet, you must avoid all foods that contain dairy products, including cheeses; all foods that contain chocolate products, including cola beverages; and any foods that contain preservatives, chemicals, flavorings, or additives.

Strictly speaking, you cannot eat in a restaurant—especially one with a salad bar or one which serves potato salad or any salad that might contain the preservative *bisulfite* that keeps such salads fresh. You cannot be certain that the restaurant doesn't use additives. Most commercially-prepared foods cannot be eaten because they contain chemicals, flavorings, or preservatives.

Eggs are not milk and may be eaten. Margarine is allowed if it is the brand specified in the salicylate additive diet in Appendix A.

Technically, you must check the label, the brand name, and the ingredient list of everything you wish to eat. Then you must cross-check it with the diet lists in Appendix A. Then you can decide whether you should eat the food. When in doubt, *do not* eat it.

Remember—at this stage you are trying to find out if foods give you symptoms by the process of eliminating combinations of foods. Later, you will find out *which* food is responsible by putting them back into your diet one at a time.

Dairy-Chocolate-Corn-Salicylate Additive Diet

For this diet you should avoid all the foods listed above, as well as corn products such as corn oil, corn meal, corn syrup, and corn starch. Corn syrup is the most difficult to avoid because it is used as a sweetener in so many foods.

ADHERE STRICTLY TO YOUR DIET

The lists in Appendix A will tell you exactly what to eat and what to avoid. They provide complete and detailed information. There are many hidden sources of these substances. For example, any food that has *caseinate* in it must be eliminated by those who are avoiding milk, cheeses, and yoghurt. Many non-dairy creamers also contain caseinate, which is derived from milk products. Likewise, cola beverages must be avoided by those who are avoiding chocolate. There are natural foods which happen to contain members of the salicylate family, and although the foods are unprocessed they must be avoided by those on this diet.

Not all foods are listed. Some haven't been tested. If the food is not listed, don't eat it.

As you read the lists you may notice inconsistencies, such as the fact that grapefruit is allowed on the salicylate additive diet while an orange is not. In such instances you must trust the accuracy of the lists. Scientific studies have shown that they are correct to the best of our ability.

MENU PLAN METHOD

For practical purposes, the easiest method of adhering to the General Elimination Diet is to use the menu plan method. You would need one menu for the dairy-chocolate-salicylate additive diet and another for the dairy-corn-chocolate-salicylate additive diet. Both menus are described on the following pages. Each has five breakfasts, five lunches, and five dinners. You do not have to follow it exactly (for example, you can eat the same breakfast and different lunches, or vice versa).

Diet Plan for Dairy-Chocolate-Salicylate Additive Diet

Breakfast

Pineapple juice	Fresh banana	Pineapple juice
Oatmeal	Hard cooked eggs	Oatmeal
Toast (white/whole wheat)	Toast (white/whole wheat)	Toast (white/whole wheat)
Margarine*	Margarine*	Margarine*

Fresh grapefruit	Fresh banana
Puffed wheat	Puffed rice
Toast (white/whole wheat)	Hard cooked egg
Margarine*	Toast (white/whole wheat)
	Margarine*

Lunch

Canadian bacon	Roast turkey sand-	*Aunt Jemima*
English muffin	wich w/ lettuce &	waffles w/ honey
Margarine*	mayonnaise	Margarine*
Carrot & celery	Carrot & celery	Canadian bacon
sticks	sticks	Fresh grapefruit
Canned pears	Fresh grapefruit	

Roast beef sand-	Baked ham sand-
wich w/ lettuce &	wich w/ lettuce &
mayonnaise	mayonnaise
Hard cooked egg	Carrot & celery
Canned pineapple	sticks
Seven-Up	Canned pineapple
	Seven-Up

* Use either *Willow Run* margarine (available in some health food stores), or you may substitute honey to sweeten toast or cooked vegetables.

Diet Plan for Dairy-Chocolate-Salicylate Additive Diet

Dinner

Lettuce salad
w/ mayonnaise
or lemon
Plain roast turkey
Carrots w/
margarine*
Rice w/ margarine*
Bread (white/whole
wheat) w/
margarine*
Fresh banana

Lettuce salad w/
mayonnaise or
lemon
Plain breast of
chicken
Mashed potato &
peas w/
margarine*
Bread (white/whole
wheat) w/
margarine*

Plain sliced roast
beef
Mashed potato &
asparagus w/
margarine*
Bread (white/whole
wheat) w/
margarine*
Canned pears

Lettuce salad w/
mayonnaise or
lemon
Plain baked ham
Corn & mashed
potato w/
margarine*
Bread (white/whole
wheat) w/
margarine*
Canned pears

Lettuce salad w/
mayonnaise or
lemon
Baked pork chops
Rice & green beans
w/ margarine*
Canned pineapple

* Use either Willow Run margarine (available in some health food stores), or
you may substitute honey to sweeten toast or cooked vegetables.

   The menu plan for the dairy-corn-chocolate-salicylate additive diet on pages 40 and 41 removes all traces of corn products.
It is difficult and rigorous. After reading it and observing its
difficulty for yourself, you may want to know if you can do
one food at a time. The answer is yes. You may do one food
at a time, but you must keep in mind the disadvantages of
eliminating one food at a time. You might not recognize the
fact that you have food allergy if you are allergic to combinations
of foods, and you may spend many months avoiding various
foods, only to learn that food allergy is not a significant cause
of your poor health.
   If you cannot find commercial bread without milk, corn, or
additives, you should use rice cakes (check the label) or make
your own bread according to the following recipe.

Oatmeal Bread

1 cup rolled oats
1 cup hot water
¼ cup pure maple syrup or
   honey
¼ teaspoon salt
2 eggs
¼ teaspoon baking soda
3 teaspoons baking
   powder (corn-free)

Mix oats and hot water. Let stand for 5 minutes. Stir in honey,
eggs, salt. Add baking soda and baking powder. Mix well. Turn
into 9″ × 5″ loaf pan. Let stand for 20 minutes in a warm place.
Bake at 350° F for 45 minutes.

   When making quick breads (see Appendix C), use fruit juice
in place of milk or water. Add 1 tablespoon of extra oil (not
corn oil!) to the recipe.
   For a beverage, you may use water, coffee, or pure fruit juice
(no corn syrup!).
   Remember that table salt may contain corn, so it's best to
use pickling salt.

If this diet seems like too much trouble to you, your doctor can prescribe an artificial, non-allergenic preparation such as *Vivonex*. *Vivonex* is completely nutritious, and you won't have to think about what you are eating. *Vivonex* comes in packets of powder that are mixed with water. However, you should not use the flavored variety, and the unflavored is not so tasty. For most people, the menu plan is a more satisfying way of adhering to the diet.

As you can see in Appendix A where each diet is explained in full, the salicylate additive diet is complex. In fact, pills are suspect because *all* medication (including vitamins) contains additives as well as the active ingredient. These substances, harmless to most people, keep the active ingredient stable, help the body to absorb the active ingredient, or color the tablet for identification. There are eight categories of substances used in pills—from fillers to binders to flavorings—to name just a few. For this reason you should take as little medication as possible when following these diets.

If you must take medication for a particular health problem, you should continue taking the medication. But you must compensate by doing a super job avoiding the other foods.

Do not discontinue any medication for the three-week test diet unless your doctor approves. Tell him the diet is only a three-week test so he doesn't think you are planning to stop his medication forever.

If you are taking medication for your allergy symptoms, continue to use it while you follow the General Elimination Diet. You may think that this will hopelessly confuse you and that you won't know whether it is the diet or the medicine that helped, but in Chapter 5 you will learn the secret of how to distinguish between the two.

If a food or food product is not listed on the sheet but pertains to your diet, it means that no one knows about it. In the United States there is a limited amount of money allocated for medical research. Because the bulk of it goes to the study of life-threatening diseases, there are foods that doctors cannot classify. In every medical specialty there are diseases for which we know a moderate amount, for which we know a little, and for which we don't know anything. We do know a lot about food allergy. We don't know every last detail about every food, but we know more than enough to find answers.

Diet Plan for Dairy-Corn-Chocolate-Salicylate Additive Diet

Breakfast

Pineapple juice
  (unsweetened)
Oatmeal
Toast (oatmeal
  bread) & honey
Margarine*

Pineapple juice
  (unsweetened)
Oatmeal
Toast (oatmeal
  bread) & honey
Margarine*

Fresh banana
Puffed rice
Hard cooked egg
Toast (oatmeal
  bread) & honey
Margarine*

Fresh grapefruit
Puffed wheat
Toast (oatmeal
  bread) & honey
Margarine*

Fresh banana
Hard cooked eggs
Toast (oatmeal
  bread) & honey
Margarine*

Lunch

Canadian bacon
  (uncured)
Carrot & celery
  sticks
Canned pears
  (unsweetened or
  in a juice
  concentrate)

Baked ham sand-
  wich (uncured) w/
  lettuce &
  mayonnaise
Carrot & celery
  sticks
Canned pineapple
  (unsweetened)

Aunt Jemima
  waffles w/ honey
Canadian bacon
  (uncured)
Fresh grapefruit

Roast beef
  sandwich w/
  lettuce &
  mayonnaise
Hard cooked egg
Canned pineapple
  (unsweetened)

Roast turkey
  sandwich w/
  lettuce &
  mayonnaise
Carrot & celery
  sticks
Fresh grapefruit

* Use either *Willow Run* margarine (available in some health food stores), or you may substitute honey to sweeten toast or cooked vegetables.

Diet Plan for Dairy-Corn-Chocolate-Salicylate Additive Diet

Dinner

Lettuce salad w/
mayonnaise or
lemon
Plain roast turkey
Carrots w/
margarine*
or honey
Rice w/ margarine*
Oatmeal bread
Fresh banana

Plain sliced roast
beef
Mashed potato &
asparagus
w/ margarine*
Oatmeal bread
Canned pears
(unsweetened or
in a juice
concentrate)

Lettuce salad w/
mayonnaise or
lemon
Plain breast of
chicken
Mashed potato &
peas w/
margarine*
Oatmeal bread &
honey

Lettuce salad w/
mayonnaise or
lemon
Plain baked ham
(uncured)
Mashed potato
Oatmeal bread
Canned pears
(unsweetened
or in a juice
concentrate)

Lettuce salad w/
mayonnaise or
lemon
Baked pork chops
Rice & green beans
w/ margarine*
Canned pineapple
(unsweetened)

* Use either *Willow Run* margarine (available in some health food stores), or
you may substitute honey to sweeten toast or cooked vegetables.

Do some detective work. Read labels. Check lists. Figure out what to eat and what not to eat. Don't accept my lists at face value because manufacturers can change how they make their product and transform a food that was once acceptable into one that is no longer agreeable. (See Appendix G for a list of major U.S. food manufacturers you might want to contact if you have any questions about a particular product.)

If you'd like more specific instructions, make an appointment with a registered dietician. These professionals are well-trained to help. They can devise a complete, balanced, and nutritious menu plan, like the one in Appendix B. This will specify brand names, serving size, and total calories. (Ordinarily, at this point such a specific diet is not required.)

It is virtually impossible to adhere to a General Elimination Diet with no errors. If you do make a mistake because you couldn't help it or did not know, keep going. Don't give up. You are not finding a specific food at this point. You are finding out whether food allergy is causing your health problem and to what extent. *A few* inadvertent mistakes won't confuse you.

A WORD ABOUT INFANTS AND CHILDREN

Infants and children must use *Nutramigen* or *Meat Base Formula* during the three-week test to replace milk. Soy products (which are the usual substitute for milk) can be allergenic and must be avoided. You should consult with your doctor beforehand, but going without milk products for three weeks is not dangerous to an infant's health, as long as the rest of the diet is well-balanced. From an overall health point of view, if milk is responsible for chronic respiratory, gastrointestinal, or another disease, then there is more harm from its continued ingestion than from its elimination.

5

Sticking To Your Diet

Although Samantha experienced recurring headaches that no one could heal, she was reluctant to undertake a General Elimination Diet. "I couldn't eat celery and water for the rest of my life!" she exclaimed to her friends. Despite her foreboding about the outcome, however, she summoned up her courage and followed the diet. Her headaches stopped. The allergenic food turned out to be wine, but Samantha's story ended happily. She found that as long as she limited her intake to no more than two glasses a week, she could drink wine without experiencing symptoms. On the few occasions she overdid it, she thought it was worth it. "At least I know that I don't have a new disease," she said. "And I can control it."

Sticking to a General Elimination Diet is the hardest part of the hunt for hidden food allergy, but you can do it! You may not enjoy it, but the payoff will be worth the effort.

Remember, this diet does not mean you should avoid one food per day. It does not mean eliminating one food one week and another food another week. It means that *all* the foods must be excluded for the *entire* three-week period. You must completely eliminate them from your body.

Sticking to the diet is a big pain. You know it, and I know it. There is nothing that can be said to convince you otherwise.

No one wants to be told that he has to diet—I wouldn't like it any more than you do!

On the other hand, if there was a way that allergy treatment could help you, you would want to know about it. If allergic reactions are responsible for a *significant* portion of your ill health, you will feel better if you find out about it and obtain the proper treatment. If not, you shouldn't waste your time on allergy treatment. Fortunately, the General Elimination Diet tells you precisely whether food allergy is a significant problem.

As soon as I mention the diet, people look desperately for another approach. You wouldn't believe the strange things I've seen some individuals do in order to avoid a General Elimination Diet, even though the diet would answer their questions. Three weeks seems like a long time when you cannot eat *what* you want *when* you want it.

Some health-conscious people worry about the lack of vitamins, calcium, and other minerals. If a person has followed a reasonable diet before, three weeks is not long enough for bones to break, hair to fall out, or scurvy to develop. If there are special considerations or you feel you'd like a second opinion, make an appointment with a Registered Dietician. Most are listed in the Yellow Pages, and when you call for an appointment ask if they are Registered Dieticians. There are health care providers who give dietary advice, such as nutritionists, weight specialists, and diet counselors, but Registered Dieticians have the "something extra" that I consider so important. They are certified by the American Dietetic Association as Registered Dieticians (R.D.). Certification requires a bachelor's degree from a college, plus a minimum of nine months to a year of supervised internship or approved clinical experience before they are allowed to take their qualifying examination. As in allergy, superior ability comes from a supervised internship or approved clinical experience in which qualified and experienced instructors point out and correct mistakes on the job, thus preparing the dietician to help you. (In some states, there are Licensed Clinical Nutritionists who have the qualifications of Registered Dieticians.)

Many patients ask for recipes and substitutes for the foods they will be avoiding on a General Elimination Diet. It's a good idea, but you should wait until the treatment phase for this.

You will have a hard enough time avoiding the foods without complicating your life by preparing dozens of special recipes. If the *test* becomes a *treatment*, then it is worth looking for substitutes. For now, however, you should concentrate on avoidance.

BEGINNING YOUR DIET

Choose three convenient weeks to do the diet. Don't begin it when relatives are coming in from out of town. Don't try to do it on a vacation. Don't do it at holiday time. But don't make all sorts of lame excuses to put it off forever, either. Get it over with!

If you make an inadvertent error on the diet because you did not know about a food or forgot about the diet, keep going. Don't start again or give up. Strictly speaking, you cannot eat outside of your house because you never know for sure what you are getting. The waiter may pretend to know that the foods don't contain preservatives or flavorings or corn byproducts, but only the chef knows for sure. And often even he doesn't know because he took the product out of a can or box.

Labels are untrustworthy. Manufacturers can change the ingredient mix and not change the label. You have to realize that there will be limitations. Just do the best you can.

Some people (or maybe I should say most people) become sorely discouraged as they go along. They want to stop eating the foods and feel better the next day, just as they would if they were experiencing immediate-type food allergy reactions. I, too, wish it would happen so fast, but it doesn't. We are dealing with delayed-type reactions here, and it can take the entire three weeks to find the answer. If it was the immediate-type reaction, you wouldn't need me, this book, or an allergist!

Sometimes people feel worse in the middle of the three weeks. This is not a bad sign. Keep on going. There are several theories about why individuals sometimes get worse before getting better. I've read the theories, but they are not proven to my satisfaction so I won't repeat them. It's not crucial to know why it happens. As long as you are aware that you may feel worse for a few days, you won't let it deter you from finishing the job you set out to do. If any symptoms occur that are different from your usual ones, see your doctor immediately.

HAVING SECOND THOUGHTS

At some point in the middle of the diet patients may have second thoughts.

•Maybe this problem is just in my head, like they say.

•Maybe this diet is a complete waste of time.

•I'd rather live with the symptoms.

•I should have done the new blood test that everyone is talking about instead of this stupid diet!

Patients are often told by their doctors that certain symptoms are in their heads. This happens when their doctors cannot detect a specific malady like cancer or diabetes. In comparison to these diseases, allergy seems like a trivial annoyance. Another situation in which patients are told their symptoms are in their head occurs when a doctor has been taught that allergy is due to emotional problems. In both cases, the attitude does a disservice to the patient.

Allergies are chronic debilitating illnesses. It's true that patients rarely die from allergies, but many allergies are so uncomfortable that people cannot function at their fullest potential. You shouldn't blame every health problem on allergy, nor should you minimize the capacity for allergy to cause a number of problems.

As for the relationship between allergy and emotions, it is not cause-and-effect. If it were, executives with high blood pressure or ulcers from being under stress would be sneezing instead! On the contrary, feeling tired and functioning below potential make people upset. Allergy can actually provoke emotional problems when an individual becomes frustrated knowing that he is not performing as well as he could.

You mustn't allow others to speculate that your problem is "all in your head." You should find out the truth. At the end of a three-week General Elimination Diet, you will have a definite answer about food allergy and can stop listening to idle chatter. It's not a waste of time to find out what ails you. If it turns out that food allergy is not your problem, you won't have to watch what you eat.

People who wish to live with their allergy symptoms are not uncommon. Often the symptoms are not life-threatening. However, that is a decision you should reserve for the treatment stage, not for the investigative stage.

Think of it this way. What if you discover that your symptoms could be cured by not eating chocolate candy? No matter how insignificant the symptoms, maybe it would be worth giving up chocolate. Maybe it wouldn't. At least if you know what is causing the problem, you have a choice. If you don't know, you are at the mercy of whatever is making you feel ill.

BLOOD TESTS FOR ALLERGY

There are three blood tests for allergy. Although patients often ask for the newest one, none of the tests is truly new. The most recent one was invented in 1968. There are different ways of performing these tests, some of which are novel, but the basic tests are the same three that have been around for twenty to thirty years.

The three types of tests can be categorized by the substance that is being measured. In other words, each one measures the function of a particular aspect of the allergy-immune system. Different companies, researchers, doctors, and university laboratories have devised different ways of measuring the same three aspects of the allergy-immune system. You could think of it as an attempt to measure the number of automobiles that pass an intersection on a given day. You could count them with your fingers and toes. You could use an abacus. You could keep a record with a calculator. Or you could purchase an advanced computer for the job. No matter how you did it, you'd still get the same result.

Another fact you must keep in mind is that "new" is not necessarily "better." When the word *new* is prominently advertised for a test or displayed on a package or label, our gullible minds leap to the conclusion that the test or product is better. This is especially true when an "expert" makes the claim. A classic (forgive the pun) example was the mistake the Coca Cola Company made when it brought out *new* Coke in 1985. The uproar from loyal *old* Coke fans sent the Coca Cola Board of

Directors scurrying to their conference room, where they quickly voted to continue selling *old Coke* (now called *Classic Coke*). There are many examples of "new" gone awry, especially in the field of medicine, where new theories and treatments are praised when they are first developed but often turn out to be of no value. From the use of leeches in the sixteenth century, to the drug *thalidomide* which caused phocomelia (congenitally absent arms) in newborns in the twentieth century, there is a rogues' gallery of snake oils and amulets that have failed to live up to their promises.

Nowhere is this more true than for the food allergy blood tests. The three types of blood tests are described below so that you will understand them.

Cytotoxic Test

In the cytotoxic test, a technician takes white cells from a person's blood and places them in a petri dish. Then he adds unmetabolized (uneaten) food to each dish, and observes whether the cell breaks. If it does, the person is said to be allergic. If you believe that adding food to a suspension of white cells can determine whether a person is allergic to a food, then you should pay special attention to this section.

The first problem with cytotoxic tests is that the wrong form of food is used to do the tests. In order for the body to absorb a food, the natural food must be metabolized (or broken down) into byproducts so it can get into the bloodstream. The byproducts of foods that are absorbed into the body are not the same as the natural food in the mouth. Although the byproducts of food are causing the reactions, it is the natural and unmetabolized form of food that is used for the testing. The reason why no one uses byproducts of foods is that no company manufactures partially digested byproducts that could be used for testing.

The second problem with cytotoxic testing is that many things can kill white cells. Even if you leave the cells alone, they will die.

Third, although the cytotoxic test is usually advertised as new and is sometimes called by a different name, such as FICA test (Food Immune Complex Assay), it was conceived over thirty years ago in the early 1950's by a Dr. Black and popularized by a Dr. Bryan. Cytotoxic tests have been thoroughly investigated using controlled studies, and there is no consistency to them. On one day a natural undigested food will kill cells; on another day it will not.

Fourth, the cytotoxic test does not take into account the effects of combinations of foods.

Fifth, it does not take into account whether the food is cooked, uncooked, pasteurized, frozen, or otherwise processed in a way that can alter the food.

Sixth, there is no medical school, university laboratory, or licensed laboratory that I know of in the United States that does cytotoxic tests. The only places I know that do them are certain doctors' offices. And to my knowledge, none of the doctors are Type I trained allergists.

Histamine Release Test

The second type of blood test is called the histamine release test, developed in the mid 1960s. To measure histamine release, a technician adds a food extract to white cells that have been taken from the bloodstream, but instead of looking at the cell and relying on human judgment to decide whether the cell is broken, he measures the chemical known as histamine. If histamine comes out of the cell, the test is said to be positive. The measurements of histamine are accurate, but the proponents of this test have not been able to show that if a white cell releases histamine, then the person reacts adversely to the food when he eats it. In other words, no one has shown a cause-and-effect relationship.

Scientists have performed the test many times and have not been able to find a relationship between histamine release and the ingestion of food. In fact, it is not quite clear what the histamine release means.

I tell the following story to illustrate that there must be a correlation between what a test says and what is actually occurring in the human body. The story goes like this. If someone came to my office with a broken arm and if I tested and found that the person was allergic to grass pollen, would that mean that their allergy to grasses had caused their broken arm? Obviously, the answer is an emphatic *no*. Grass pollen allergy and a broken arm are two different illnesses. The two conditions have nothing to do with each other, and a positive x-ray showing a broken arm does not mean that the person is allergic to grasses. Similarly, a positive test for grass pollen does not indicate a broken arm.

It is the same situation with histamine release. When a food that released histamine is fed to a patient, the patient often experiences no symptoms whatsoever. Conversely, many patients experience symptoms after eating foods that did not trigger histamine release.

RAST-Type Tests

RAST tests are the latest rage in diagnosis. Each company has created a name to distinguish its RAST-type test from the others. The common ones are RAST, FAST, MAST, and ELISA. The idea behind them is to save patients from the supposed pain of skin testing. The RAST-type blood tests and skin tests both measure IgE antibody. As you already know from an earlier chapter, too much IgE causes an overreaction and produces hypersensitivity to things that ordinarily wouldn't bother anyone.

Although both the blood and skin tests measure IgE antibody, there are two problems with the RAST-type tests. The first is that they are slightly less accurate than skin tests. Most of the IgE in the body is attached to the mast cells in the skin. It's in the skin surface of the nose, the surface of the eyes and sinuses, the surface of the airways in the lung, and the surface of the gastrointestinal tract. Very little floats in the blood. Furthermore, of the IgE that is in the blood, most of it is attached to a cell called a Basophil. Hardly any IgE floats freely, where it can be measured by the RAST-type tests. Since the allergic reactions occur in the skin and not in the blood, perhaps this is why the skin tests are more accurate.

The second problem with RAST-type blood tests is that they cost so much more—often three to five times as much. For this reason, for the greater accuracy of skin tests, and because the results of skin tests are available within fifteen minutes, trained allergists prefer to do them. The argument concerning the pain of skin tests is false. Allergists don't dig huge needles into the skin. There is no bleeding when the common scratch test is done because the scratch is so superficial. In the case of children or people in whom it is difficult to draw blood, the procedure for obtaining a sample of blood can be much more uncomfortable and painful than any of the skin tests.

GENERAL COMMENTS ABOUT THE BLOOD TESTS

The advertisements for blood tests present glowing claims. Unfortunately, controlled experiments do not support the claims. Scientifically-done experiments show that the blood test accuracy rate is in the vicinity of 20%. When I first learned this statistic, it didn't make any sense. Flipping a coin is 50% accurate, and I thought a scientific test should at least be better than flipping coins! The reason for the poor accuracy is that the tests can be both falsely positive and falsely negative. In a false positive test, the individual does not react when he eats the food. In a false negative test, the individual does react when he eats the food, even though the test predicted that there would be no reaction.

As if it wasn't confusing enough, there is a cumulative factor involved in producing the actual symptoms. The degree of susceptibility in each individual is different. Some people are so sensitive that a single bite of chocolate will trigger a reaction. Others must eat ten bites before they become ill. Some might have to ingest two pounds of chocolate before exceeding their threshold. If a person is susceptible at a level of two pounds, he might never know he was allergic because so few people can eat two pounds in one sitting! This can be illustrated by a mathematical equation:

food allergy *symptoms* = susceptibility + ingestion of food

The more susceptible the person, the less food he must ingest to provoke symptoms. The less susceptible the person, the more he must ingest. The blood tests don't evaluate how much a person eats, and do not indicate whether allergy to the food provokes the bothersome symptom.

When scientists invent a perfect way of making the blood tests accurate at pinpointing an allergenic food, the tests will still be deficient because they will ignore the critical factors of exposure, quantity, and relevance to the person's major problem.

ARE YOU SURE YOU'RE ALLERGIC?

Another factor that contributes to widespread misunderstanding about food allergy is that there are several other classifications of adverse reactions to foods that may mimic allergies. For example, some individuals lack an enzyme that digests the sugar in milk. The sugar is called lactose, and the enzyme that digests it is called lactase. In the absence of lactase, a person who ingests milk will experience cramps, stomachaches and diarrhea (see Appendix F). Another example is that of people with gallbladder disease. In these individuals, greasy foods will provoke abdominal cramps. There are food idiosyncrasies, food poisonings, and food enzyme disturbances that cause symptoms but are *not* allergic conditions. Below is a list of types of food reactions.

- Allergy—A reaction to foods due to excess levels of IgE antibody.

- Poisoning—A reaction to foods that contain harmful bacteria or their toxic byproducts.

- Metabolic—A reaction usually due to an enzyme deficiency and an inability to digest a food properly, such as the reaction to milk due to deficiency of the digestive enzyme lactase.

- Pharmacologic—A reaction to a food that contains a chemical that can provoke symptoms, such as the "jitters" from the caffeine in coffee.

SUMMING UP

The moral to this story is simple. You are looking for hidden food allergy. To do so, you must stay on your General Elimination Diet. It is the 100% accurate method of discovering a hidden food allergy and learning to what extent the hidden food allergy is responsible for your problems. You may not be able to stick to the diet 100% but, remember, *you are not attempting to pinpoint a specific food at this time.* You are learning whether you have food allergy and to what extent food allergy causes your symptoms. If you can only do the diet 90%, you will still be able to judge the results, so don't let an inadvertent mistake stop you. Keep going. Ordinarily, one or two mistakes won't change the results.

I don't want you to become discouraged by a few mistakes. I want you to learn the facts about the possible role that food allergy plays in causing you to feel ill or function poorly. If food allergy is the key to good health in your case, I want you to know it.

During these three weeks, you will not go hungry. You can eat as much as you want of the allowed foods. You may even gain weight. You may yearn for a particular food, but you won't starve.

Don't waste time looking for shortcuts. Don't make the mistake of doing a Specific Elimination Diet or paying for dozens of inaccurate skin or blood tests when you may not even have food allergy. Stay on the right path. You will be amply rewarded for your effort.

Remember, no slip-ups! At this stage the General Elimination Diet is a *test*, not a treatment.

6
Evaluating the Results

William suffered from severe gastrointestinal pain, fatigue, and irritability. He was snapping at his wife and angry at his boss. He was so unhappy that he was even considering early retirement. On his doctor's advice he began the General Elimination Diet to determine whether foods were causing his gastrointestinal symptoms. Within a week he began to feel better. His attitude at work changed, and he was pleasant at home. However, his stomach symptoms persisted. William had discovered that foods were responsible for his malaise, but that he would have to look elsewhere to find out what caused his gastrointestinal problem.

Now that you have reached the end of the three weeks, give yourself a pat on the back. You did it! You avoided the suspect foods, and you cleansed your body. You invested three weeks of your time, and you can reap the reward for a job well done.

Your reward is that you will discover whether food allergy has caused your problems and to what extent it caused them. Here's how to find out. Ask yourself the following two questions.

•How did I feel during the final week of my three-week diet? Forget the first two weeks. They don't count. They were meant to clean you out. Think only of the third week.

•Overall, do I feel 80% better, 50% better, or 10% better than before I started the diet?

BACK TO THE FOOD ALLERGY BASELINE

Now take out your Food Allergy Baseline, on which you wrote down your symptoms. At the top of the page write your answer to the second question. By what percentage did you improve during the third week of the diet compared to before you started the diet? Then, item by item, go down the list. In Column 5 write down how many days each symptom occurred during the final seven days of the diet. Did it occur five of those last seven days (5/7), two of them (2/7), or none (0/7)? In Column 6 decide how much better that particular symptom was. Did it improve 50%, 10%, or 2%?

For the next step you must decide whether your symptom improved on its own or improved because of the diet. If your symptoms have a history of fluctuating, you could have started the diet at precisely the time when you would have improved naturally. If your experience has been that a symptom can go away by itself for two months, then you cannot conclude from three weeks of dieting that the diet helped. Improvement could have just been a coincidence. In order to be positive that the diet had helped, you would have to remain on the diet for two and a half months so you would not be *tricked* into thinking it had worked.

Next, look at Column 4 on your sheet. It tells you how long each symptom could go away with no intervention. Check either Column 7 or Column 8, depending on whether the symptom could have improved on its own or not.

For example, if Column 4 states that in the past your symptom occurred every day, and Column 5 states that after the diet it dropped to one day of the past seven, this constitutes a significant change in the pattern. It indicates that food allergy is the answer to your problem. On the other hand, if Column 4 states that you used to have symptoms two out of every seven days, and Column 5 states that after the diet you had symptoms one out of every seven days, this is not a significant change. You would have to be symptom-free every day of the past week to conclude that there was meaningful improvement.

Some people are amazed that it could take three weeks to clear a food from their bodies. They are convinced that foods leave their bodies within a few hours after eating, and that they should feel better the next day. This pattern occurs only when the reaction is of the immediate-type, such as the immediate reaction to eggs, nuts, seafood, or fruit.

For the delayed-type reaction, the pattern is quite different. Some of the breakdown products of foods are small molecules that can bind to cells in the body. The most carefully-studied example of this occurs in penicillin allergy, where one of the breakdown products of penicillin attaches to red blood cells and can remain in the bloodstream for the four-month life of the red blood cell. If the individual is allergic to that particular breakdown product, it would take four months for him to recover. This is an extreme example, but it illustrates the fact that delayed reactions can take several weeks to subside.

Recognizing that an allergic reaction has subsided takes time. The allergenic food must be eliminated, the reaction stopped, and the healing process completed before you will be aware that you feel better. You can't rush Mother Nature!

NEED MORE TIME?

There are virtually no situations in which more than three weeks of dieting is needed in order to decide whether you have food allergy. However, there is one that I feel I should mention: I hesitate to discuss it because there is no scientific evidence that it is true. But there is a popular theory that hidden food allergy is responsible for difficulty with losing weight. Although there are no facts to support this claim, people who are having a hard time losing weight want to explore any possibility. There is no harm in experimenting.

In such a case, the supposed food allergy may not show up as fast as three weeks, so you might have to stay on the diet for up to five weeks. I would prefer to have scientific proof before recommending this as a possible method to help lose weight, but here, too, you can test the theory in your own body by following the procedure outlined in this book.

If you use medication for symptomatic relief of allergies while you are on the diet, you will not know whether your improvement is due to the medication or the diet. In this situation, continue the diet and *under your doctor's direction* stop the medication. Most drugs leave the body within two or three days. If you continue to feel better after discontinuing the medication, you may conclude that the diet helped.

THE MOMENT OF TRUTH

Now you are ready for one of the most important steps of all. This, in fact, is the moment of truth.

Read over your list of symptoms again. Did the most bothersome symptoms (the ones you previously starred) improve? If not, there is no point in continuing. You have just shown that eliminating potentially allergenic foods from your body did not alter the symptoms that were most bothersome.

If minor health problems changed, you may want to continue the investigation to find the offending food, but at least you know that food allergy is responsible for only minor symptoms. You have to decide whether the symptoms are worth bothering about.

If your most bothersome symptom did not improve and you are still convinced that foods are making you ill, you may be right. The foods you have been eating during the elimination phase may be the true offenders. In that case, do the General Elimination Diet in reverse. Eat only those foods you have avoided for the previous three weeks. If you remain ill, it is time to abandon the idea that food allergy is responsible for your symptoms. There is no point in hoping that the solution to your health problem is as simple as an allergy to foods, when you have just proven that in your case food is not the answer. Accepting this answer may be difficult, but accept it we must!

FACING UP TO THE TRUTH

At this point the candidate for food allergy must often face up to a most painful realization. If the elimination diet did not help and the reverse elimination diet did not help, then he must face the fact that food allergy is not to blame for his problem. He will have to search for another solution, whether it be physical or psychological.

Learning that food allergy is not the answer to a patient's problem is a difficult outcome to accept. At the outset my patients and I are filled with hope that we will nail the problem that plagues them and is causing their poor health. As an allergist I have a privileged position that cushions my disappointment. I can take comfort in the fact that my job was to prove that food allergy is or is not a factor. The patient, on the other hand, must live with the outcome. I console myself with the fact that I saved them from needless tests, useless diets, or false hopes that food allergy would be a miracle cure.

For the patient, I become another doctor in a long line of physicians who say they don't know what is causing their illness. I can't describe how discouraging it is for the patient, but I'd like to remind you that it's better not to do anything for a health problem until you know what to do than to do something just for the sake of keeping busy. When an individual utilizes a treatment that has proven to be of little value, he is merely deluding himself. He doesn't accomplish anything, and may be putting off the search for what could really help.

MOVING ON

For those lucky enough to have improved, you must answer one more question before going on to the next chapter.

•Did you improve *enough* to be worth going through the next phase of finding out which food is the culprit?

If you are 100% better, the answer is a resounding *yes*. Once you identify the allergenic food, you will be very relieved. You will function better. You will live better. It's worth whatever effort it takes.

On the other hand, if you are only 10% better, it may not be worth your while to spend time searching for the offending food. When you do find it, you will be 90% short of your goal of achieving complete relief.

There are instances where a person chooses to work on the 10% because there is no other possible help for his condition. He decides that 10% relief is better than nothing. As long as such a person knows that he is working towards partial relief and not towards the cure, this is perfectly acceptable.

I don't want readers of this book to be guilty of the common error of getting their priorities backwards. Don't spend inordinate amounts of time and money working on 10% of a problem while the 90% factor goes unrecognized and untreated. Keep your priorities clearly in focus. I have consulted many individuals who became sidetracked from their original problem and spent years treating symptoms that were not interfering with their health, their lifestyle, or their enjoyment of life.

7

Finding the Culprit

Michael was so proud that he had stuck to his diet for three weeks (with no slip-ups) that he went out to celebrate—prematurely. He ordered an extra large pizza at his favorite shop. Then he went next door for a double scoop of chocolate ice cream smothered in hot fudge. Needless to say, his symptoms returned. He had no idea what food had made him so sick.

Finding the specific food to which you are allergic is the step everyone wants to do first. Nothing I say or do will change this. Nevertheless, I am stubbornly opposed to any attempt to pinpoint a specific food until it is known for sure that food allergy is a significant problem.

No one would undertake a costly analysis for cardiac surgery unless they had a clue that they suffered from heart disease. No one would consider elaborate testing for hormonal problems unless there was an indication that they suffered from hormonal disease. Yet people often begin an analysis or long-term investigation for food allergy before fully understanding whether food allergy is the source of their health problem. By following the steps outlined in this book, you have not made this mistake!

At this point you know that you have food allergy and you know that it is worth looking into. You are now ready to narrow the search.

PUTTING THE FOODS BACK

To find the specific food, you must put the foods back into your diet in a systematic way. Start with whatever food you have missed the most while being on the General Elimination Diet. Begin eating the food. It doesn't matter whether you choose a "healthy" food or a "non-healthy" food. You have earned the right to eat.

For five days in a row, continue the General Elimination Diet while you add the new food. You must eat a lot of this food. Eat more of it than you normally would. If you had stopped drinking milk and you used to have a glass a day, you should consume one and a half glasses a day for the next five days. If you avoided wheat and you used to have four slices of bread a day, you should eat six slices. Select one food at a time and eat more of it than you used to because you want to trigger a reaction. It doesn't sound like proper advice from a physician, but you understand the idea.

Eliminate the food and get better. Eat it and get sick. It proves the point both ways.

Be careful when adding foods. Allergic individuals may have immediate and strong reactions. Severe reactions can occur to foods such as nuts, shellfish, and eggs, and to chemicals such as aspirin and the chemical sulfites used in some salad bars.

When allergenic foods have been eliminated, their reintroduction can result in reactions sooner and sometimes harder than when the person was eating them on a regular basis.

You should add foods under a doctor's supervision, especially if you are susceptible to asthma, swelling of the throat, or any potentially life-threatening reaction. In most cases severe reactions will not occur because most of the reactions discussed in this book are the delayed-type. Still, you should be aware of the possibility.

Keep a list of what happens after you eat each food. There are three possible outcomes. Either you'll react, you won't react, or you won't be able to tell whether you reacted. Analyze the results. Make a chart like the one on the next page. Call it the Provocative Challenge Results. Post it in the kitchen where you can see it. At the end of each five-day period, record the results.

Provocative Challenge Results

OK Foods	Not OK Foods	Don't Know

COMPLETING THE CHART

OK Foods means that during the five days in which you added a particular food to your General Elimination Diet and were diligent about eating more of it than you usually would, your symptoms did not appear. When you flood the system this way, five days is long enough to provoke the symptoms. If you remained well while eating substantial amounts of this food, it means that the food is not a significant contributor to your health problem. It means that you can eat the food without fear, guilt, or worry.

Write the food in the OK column. Continue eating it in *usual* amounts. Choose another food and repeat the process until you have sorted all the foods in your diet into the columns on the chart.

Not OK Foods means that your symptoms occurred during the five-day period. In this case, stop eating the food and write it in this column. This food can produce unwanted symptoms, and you should not be eating it. Wait until the food has been cleared out of your system. You will know by the way you feel. Once you are better, try another food.

There is one note of caution for those of you who must avoid milk. You should obtain calcium tablets and take them regularly. Your doctor or registered dietician can tell you the correct dose.

Don't Know means that you developed symptoms during the five-day provocation period, but are not sure if they were due to the added food, a cold, or fatigue. In this case write the food down in this column. When you feel better, try it again.

ONE FOOD AT A TIME, PLEASE!

Just looking at the thousands of foods on grocery shelves leads one to believe that it would take two lifetimes to add one food at a time. As strange as it sounds, two lifetimes would be optimistic! Most stores stock at least 15,000 food items, and at five days per item it would take 75,000 days, or 205 years, to test every one. However, from a practical point of view, individuals don't eat the thousands of different foods that are available. Most individuals eat the same basic foods on a day-to-day basis. We all have a favorite drink, a favorite fruit, two or three favorite vegetables, beef, chicken, pork, and fish. Once in a while we are daring and try something new, but we generally eat the same types of meals.

In an effort to hasten the process of testing one food at a time, some patients want to eat several foods at once. Some even want to start with pizza—a combination of grains, dairy products, corn starch, tomatoes, seasonings, flavorings, vegetables, meat, and spices!

Approach the problem from a logical point of view. You must eat more pizza for five days in a row than you would ordinarily eat in one day. Some hardy individuals may welcome such an experience, and if you do not develop symptoms you will have learned about many substances at once. But remember, you must eat the same pizza every day for five days.

Now look at the other side of the coin. If you became ill, you would not know which ingredient was to blame. You have to start from the beginning, clean yourself out, and then add one food at a time.

When you add by groups, you have more to lose than you have to gain. Even ice cream is a "group" because it contains dairy products, flavorings, fruits, nuts, cookies, and candies. So think before you eat. Different brands of the same food can be made with different ingredients, so you may be able to tolerate one and not another.

You must test everything separately. You stuck to the elimination diet. You're coming down the home stretch. The worst is behind you. Be patient. Don't ruin all your hard work. End the search for hidden food allergy properly and scientifically.

There is another insurmountable problem. Foods are inadequately labelled for the allergenic patient. When a label states that the product contains "vegetable oil," for example, it could be coconut, corn, cottonseed, palm, palm kernel, peanut, rapeseed, safflower, soybean, or sunflower! Manufacturers are not legally required to specify which oil they use. To make matters worse, companies sometimes substitute oils from one batch to another, depending on price, availability, and the quality of the different oils.

Pills can contain filler, flavoring, and coloring substances in addition to the active ingredient. There are pitfalls to everything you eat, and you must ask your body to be the final judge of what you can and cannot tolerate.

If you've heard that yoghurt is not as bad as milk, or whole wheat is not as bad as bleached, or green grapes are not as bad as red, or cooked apples are not as bad as raw, you've probably heard correctly. What you didn't hear was the phrase "for me." When someone tells you that yoghurt is not as bad as milk, he should also add that this is true for him and may not necessarily be true for you.

Do not be lulled into a false sense of security by the experiences of neighbors, relatives, friends, or doctors. You are different from them. Your metabolism is different from theirs. Your body is different from theirs, and in all likelihood your symptoms are different from theirs. There is no reason to assume that what worked for them will work for you.

You invested the time and energy to stick to a General Elimination Diet. You're on the right track. Don't throw away your chance to pin down the exact cause of your problem by taking a shortcut.

Stick to your goal. Find out what is making *you* ill. Remember, one food at a time. One brand at a time. One pill at a time. One drink at a time.

8
Treating the Food Allergy

Peter was overjoyed when he discovered that ice cream, cheeses, and chocolate were at the bottom of his malaise and irritability. But when he thought about giving them up for the rest of his life, his joy turned to depression. So over the following weeks Peter experimented with his diet. He learned that he could eat ice cream once a week and ingest moderate amounts of chocolate twice a week without triggering his symptoms. He could no longer binge on ice cream and chocolate, but this was a compromise he could live with.

By the time you reach this chapter, I hope you have realized that I prefer advice that is guaranteed to give results. Such a guarantee is not always possible in many fields of medicine, but in food allergy it is. I promise you that avoiding an allergenic food will always prevent the symptoms, just as eating enough of an allergenic food will always produce the symptoms.

No one has to tell you that avoidance is the best treatment for food allergy. You may not like hearing it, but a fact is a fact. You should avoid any foods that make you sick. *Don't eat it if you are allergic to it.*

When a patient brings me a list of foods that he or she has found to be allergenic, I pray that the foods are pomegranates, kiwi fruit, and rhubarb—the kinds of foods that most people could stop eating without a moment of regret!

Unfortunately, life is not always so kind. The foods can just as easily be those the person loves to eat regularly. The situation is worse when multiple foods are involved. In that case the person may throw up his hands in despair. Some people are eager to follow the steps for diagnosis of food allergy on the assumption that they are allergic to hazelnuts, in which case they would gladly give up hazelnuts to rid themselves of their chronic health problem. But when the results are in and it turns out that they are allergic to chocolate, they say, "Wait a minute! I was willing to give up hazelnuts, but chocolate is another story." It may be impossible for chocolate lovers to believe, but chocolate is not essential to one's health!

If you are allergic to many different foods or to foods that contain essential ingredients, you should consult a registered dietician. Bring the dietician your list of forbidden foods. He will teach you how to achieve a balanced diet. He will explain what supplements you should take. In some states there are licensed nutritionists. This type of individual is also qualified to help you. Be sure to specify that you want a registered dietician or licensed nutritionist.

Nothing works better than avoidance for the treatment of food allergy, but avoidance of a food is boring, frustrating, and a restraint of personal freedom. It's depressing and (pardon the pun) distasteful.

HOW *NOT* TO HAVE YOUR CAKE (AND EAT IT, TOO!)

In most cases of food allergy you can eat as much as you want as long as you don't care how you feel. Food allergies don't usually cause life-threatening diseases. If you eat the allergenic foods, you know what you are doing. You know you are taking a calculated risk, and you know the outcome. It's a decision you will have to make for yourself.

When a food produces minor symptoms, it may not be important to avoid it. Some individuals sneeze two or three times after they eat a food, and it's really no big deal.

In certain cases, you may try small amounts of the allergenic food. Often, small amounts can be tolerated as long as you do not go overboard. Food allergy is like a bucket of water. When you pour water into a bucket, eventually the water will overflow and soak the ground. As long as the water does not spill over the top of the bucket, the ground will remain dry. Food allergy behaves in the same way. For example, an individual who is strongly allergic to peanuts might experience symptoms (overflow his bucket) after just one peanut. A moderately sensitive person would have to eat more, and a relatively non-sensitive individual might have to eat a bucketful in order to produce symptoms. This is the reason why you must eat more than usual during the challenge (or provocation) phase of the diet.

I encourage each of you to do the provocation test again to learn to what extent you can tolerate the *Not OK Foods*. This time, instead of eating more than you usually do, gradually increase the amount. Find out how much you can tolerate, and in the future keep below that limit.

Once you know the foods that are allergenic and after you experiment to find out how much you can tolerate, you will have to decide how much better you want to feel: 10%, 50%, or 100% better? The more you avoid the allergenic food, the better you will feel.

Don't Let Your Guard Down

After a period of eating small amounts of food without experiencing a reaction, you might incorrectly assume that you have outgrown your allergy. You might begin to eat as much as, or more than, ever. Under these circumstances your symptoms may reappear. When you have been gradually increasing your intake for a long time, you may assume that the recurrence of symptoms cannot be due to the original food because, you reason, you should have been feeling ill when you first started.

On the contrary, it can take time to fill your bucket to the overflow point by eating a little at a time. If this happens to you, go back to square one. Stop eating the food and see if you improve. Remember, from now on you must keep in mind that you are an individual who is subject to food allergy. You must think of food allergy when you experience symptoms. The bright spot is that you have trained yourself to diagnose and treat it.

Find Substitutes

You may make substitutions for foods. For example, try goat's milk for cow's milk. Or try soy milk. Cooked foods such as baked apples may be tolerated, while natural foods such as raw apples may not be. In some cases the natural food is acceptable and the cooked is not.

You can try anything, but be careful! Be ready to abandon the experiment if symptoms appear.

For professional advice, consult a Registered Dietician. They have been specifically trained to prepare well-rounded, healthful and satisfying diets. They can help you to find the best substitutes.

The list of families of foods in Appendix D will help you to identify foods that are related to the foods you discovered are allergenic. You can experiment with foods in the same category, but it would be safer to choose foods from unrelated categories.

Don't Be Complacent With Substitutes

As a person who is subject to hidden food allergy reactions, you must exercise caution with substitute foods. You may tolerate substitutions for a while and then become allergic to them. It sounds discouraging, but if you are alert to the possibility, you can handle it.

A classic example is when infants who are allergic to cow's milk are switched to soy milk. After a period of time they can become allergic to soy milk as well.

Free of Food Allergy Forever

One of the exciting facts about food allergy is that after a period of complete elimination, the body can sometimes tolerate the food. Although there are many theories about this, no one has explained the transformation satisfactorily, nor has anyone been able to bring the transformation about. It just happens. Sometimes the allergy goes away for months or years and sometimes it goes away forever. You will have to test your own body from time to time to learn whether you are one of the lucky ones.

Rotation Diet

An excellent method of circumventing food allergy is the rotation diet. By rotating foods in your diet so that you do not eat the same food on successive days, you can prevent the accumulation of foods in your system to the point where they can provoke symptoms. You must experiment to find out how often to rotate or whether rotation will even work for you. Rotation is not a panacea, and some individuals react to a food even if they only eat it once a year.

There is a popular notion that if you use a rotation diet you can *prevent* allergies from occurring in the first place. No one has proven that this idea is true, but many people adhere to it because it sounds plausible.

We know that allergy develops after exposure to allergenic substances, and the more you are exposed, the more likely it is that you will become allergic. Rotation reduces exposure, but does not eliminate it. Thus, a person who was destined to become allergic after one year of eating peanuts every day would become allergic after two years of eating peanuts every other day or after three years of eating peanuts every third day. And if you ate twice as many peanuts a day every other day, you would become allergic in the same one year.

Think what would happen if you did not have an allergic predisposition. You would be rotating your diet according to a complex formula for a problem that would never arise.

Traditional Treatment Can Sometimes Help

Many people have read about one or all of the three common treatments for respiratory allergy: avoidance, use of medication, and allergy injections. Medication and injections can sometimes help in food allergy cases.

Medication

Hundreds of different drugs are available for treating allergies, and each manufacturer claims that his is better than his competitor's. Admittedly, the drugs can do a wonderful job, but they have disadvantages, too. They can cause side effects such as sleepiness, the jitters, and an upset stomach. In some people, the side effects are even worse than the original disease. Another problem occurs when individuals build up a resistance to the drug and the drug stops working. A third problem that is encountered is that the drugs may not help despite the advertised claims.

The most significant problem in using medication for allergies is that no one has invented a medicine that cures allergy. The drugs may relieve the symptoms and make a person feel better, but they don't correct the underlying condition. The situation is no different from other branches of medicine. Insulin doesn't cure diabetes, but that does not mean that diabetics should not use it. As long as you are aware of the limitations of drugs, you will know what to expect and how to use them.

You may think of allergy drugs as a mechanism to keep the lid on the bucket. But they cannot reverse the underlying pathology.

There are three types of drugs which, to varying degrees, have been used in food allergy cases. They are antihistamines, bronchodilators, and *Cromolyn*. If you wish to try them for your food allergy symptoms, you should ask your doctor. In the few lucky cases in which these drugs ameliorate symptoms, the effect takes hold in a matter of days. So you don't have to use them for months to learn whether they would help you.

There are three situations in which the drugs are likely to help. When food allergy causes itching and hives, antihistamines can stop this. In those who experience coughing, wheezing, and shortness of breath (asthma), bronchodilators can help the chest symptoms. In those who have gastrointestinal symptoms, *Cromolyn* (when taken orally before the food is ingested) has been shown to prevent allergic symptoms from occurring in certain individuals.

Allergy Injections

Allergy injections do not help food allergy directly. They work indirectly, and you will have to understand what they do to see how they can help food allergy sufferers. The mechanism is interesting.

The goal of allergy injections is to force the body to make more of the IgG type of antibody as a kind of counterbalance to the excessive levels of IgE antibody that are being made in people who are allergic. There is much more to it than simply tipping a scale away from IgE toward the direction of IgG. IgG can actually block the allergy reaction from taking place. In fact, doctors have named IgG "blocking antibody."

To start an injection program, a doctor injects a serum just below the skin surface. The serum contains allergenic substances such as grass pollen, dust, or animal dander.

The method works because the cells that make IgE antibody are located in the skin surfaces, while the cells that make IgG antibody are located inside the body in the liver, lymph nodes, and spleen. Bypassing the skin surface and introducing the serum inside forces the body preferentially to make IgG instead of IgE antibody.

Once injections are started, the doctor gradually increases the dose of serum. Using the high-dose method, he would give injections once or twice a week for two and a half months to build to a maintenance dose. Since the maintenance dose can last for three to four weeks, the patient would then switch to a once-a-month schedule. After three years, injections can generally be stopped.

If a doctor uses the low-dose method, his patients would need more injections more often and for more years than with the high-dose method. In some offices the patient is required to come twice a week for six to nine months, then once a week for a few years, then every other week, and so forth. It's not right or wrong to use the low-dose versus the high-dose method because both are designed to build up the IgG to counteract the effect of the IgE, but the high-dose method requires fewer visits for fewer years.

There is variation to the above statements because each person is individual and reacts differently, but after following the high-dose method for three years, the IgG level is generally raised and the level of IgE is reduced so that the patient can discontinue his injections without a relapse in his or her symptoms.

However, experiment after experiment has shown that injections are not directly useful for food allergy. In fact, several people died when they were injected with foods. It sounds scary, and it is. There are no situations I've encountered where allergy injections *for foods* are worth the risk.

For airborne allergens the story is the opposite. The injections are safe, effective, and well worthwhile. In fact, if an individual has allergy to airborne material and foods, injections for airborne allergens can, in some cases, reduce the total allergic load on their system so that foods are more easily tolerated. This is the *indirect* effect I mentioned above.

Cortisone

I call cortisone a treatment of last resort because steroids (the general name for all brands of cortisone) can cause long-term, serious complications. Some brand names are *Prednisone, Prednisolone, Medrol, Aristocort, Decadron, Depo-Medrol, Beclomethosone, Nasalide, Vancenase, Beconase, Kenalog,* and *Funisolide.* The side effects can include weight gain, high blood pressure, ulcer, cataracts, softening of bones, and stunting of growth. There can be psychological changes. Most, but not all, of the effects occur after prolonged use. If no other treatment has helped, a doctor may have no choice but to use steroids.

Like other drugs, cortisone does not cure the underlying disease. If cortisone ultimately cured food allergy, maybe it would be worth the risk of its serious, long-term side effects. But cortisone is palliative. It's a big risk for a little reward.

Sometimes it's hard for a patient to know he is using steroids. He may have been told he was using *Medrol* and might not be aware that *Medrol* is a brand of steroid. He may have an "allergy shot" in the nose or buttocks and not know that most allergy shots in the nose or buttocks are steroids. Even nasal sprays can be steroids.

THE BEST ADVICE?

As is true in many aspects of life, the more you work towards a goal, the greater your chance of success. The same principle holds true for food allergy treatment. You must decide how far to go. Should you go all the way to achieve complete relief or part of the way to achieve partial relief? It would not make sense for you to invest enormous time and effort on a minor problem.

In economic courses in college, students learn about the Law of Diminishing Returns. This is why it is so important to find out how severe your food allergy problem is *before* .you begin to search for and treat your hidden food allergy. You must also be careful to treat food allergy only if it alleviates problems that are significant and therefore worth the effort you will have to expend.

The scientifically- and medically-best advice is not always the best advice for an individual. You should participate in the decisions about your care. Think about it from *your* point of view. Weigh the advantages and disadvantages. Calculate how much you would gain if you followed the prescribed regimen. Follow the treatment that works out best for you from an overall point of view.

If expending great effort to avoid foods results in three fewer sneezes a year, it is not worth the trouble. If avoiding several foods improves how you feel, how you function, how you behave, and how you relate to other people, then you should make avoidance of allergenic foods a way of life.

9
The Future of Food Allergy

The Jenkins family suspected that food allergy might be responsible for the chronic nasal congestion that had become a family trademark. They were eager to investigate food allergy, but their diets were aleady so complicated that no one wanted to do an elimination diet, too. Mom was on a weight-loss diet. Dad followed a low-cholesterol diet. The children were fussy eaters. And Grandma (who lived with them) had a special diet for her diabetes.

One day, Mr. Jenkins spotted an ad in the newspaper for a brand new test for food allergy. Mrs. Jenkins made an appointment. They were told that the test measured antibodies, was new, and had been used in other parts of the world. It was not, however, accepted by traditional doctors. Several thousands of dollars later, the Jenkins family was given a computer printout showing that they were as allergic to foods they rarely or never ate as to foods they ate regularly. The tests did not take into account cooking, pasteurizing, processing, or otherwise altering foods. The tests had to be double checked by an elimination diet. And, most important, the tests did not indicate whether the supposedly allergenic foods caused their chronic nasal congestion or whether the family congestion was due to the fact that they also bred dogs and had five or six puppies in the house at any one time.

In the years to come you will read of new treatments and new tests for food allergy. This is good news for all of us. The more we study, the more we learn. The more we learn, the better we can treat food allergy. Scientists welcome theories. If no one had new ideas, we would still be using Stone Age techniques to solve modern medical problems.

When you hear of a new idea, find out as much about it as you can. Ask your family doctor or your allergy doctor. Learn whether the new idea applies to you. There are many pitfalls between having an idea and turning the idea into a bona fide treatment.

People are embarrassed to ask their doctor what they think might be a "stupid" question. But you cannot afford to think this way. You are dealing with your health. You must understand as much as you can so you can make proper decisions. I have been asked hundreds and hundreds of questions, and I've never encountered a stupid one. There have been misunderstandings. There have been partial truths. There have been inflated and misleading advertising claims. There have been exaggerated newspaper and magazine articles. But I've never heard a "stupid" question.

Always remember that you do not really need a new idea in food allergy, anyway. You already know of a method that is guaranteed to give accurate answers 100% of the time, and costs practically nothing. The best you can hope for in the future is a test that is faster or easier, but nothing can be more accurate than 100%.

Most of your information will come from newspapers, magazines, television, radio, or friends. It is difficult for these sources to completely understand the technical details of medical research that make one experiment valuable and another worthless. Even doctors often argue about the significance of experimental results. You must be your own guide. You must ask yourself the following questions.

- Is the new treatment or test really better than the "tried and true" method?

- Is the new proposal much more expensive or time-consuming than the old method?

• Has the new idea been tested?

• Is the new theory faster but less accurate?

• Has the new theory been tested only by its proponents, who might have been prejudiced or might have overlooked a crucial factor in their zeal to promote their new test? Or has it been evaluated by an impartial third party?

• Do the proponents of the new proposal tell us what percentage of people achieved relief, what percentage showed no change, and what percentage felt worse?

Be wary when the strongest testimonial for an idea comes from entertainment and sports personalities, who are being paid to advertise it. Such advice is anecdotal because it is based upon their personal experience. Your body may not respond as theirs did.

You must always ask what the information or advice means for *you*. If a few highly allergic individuals become deathly ill when they eat peanuts, this doesn't mean that the government must ban peanuts for all of us.

Many times your doctor will tell you that an idea is *unproven*. You should ask him what he means. *Unproven* can mean any of the following:

• The treatment and theory were proven wrong.

• The treatment and theory were tested only by their proponents, but double blind controlled tests by an impartial third party have not yet been done. This means that we have only the prejudiced word of the promoters for how well it works.

• No one has run any kind of controlled or uncontrolled tests, which means that at this point the idea is pure supposition.

LOOKING INTO THE CRYSTAL BALL

Although predicting the future is foolhardy, I would like to make a few predictions here.

I predict that no one will invent a more accurate test than the General Elimination Diet test, followed by provocative challenge. Our bodies are too different. Our tastes in food are too different. Our other medical problems are too different. Our lifestyles are too different. Each of these factors determines how foods affect us, and only your own body can tell you how a food will affect *you*.

I predict that no one will invent a more guaranteed method of stopping food allergy reactions than avoiding the food. You will hear claims for new techniques, and in some cases the new technique will help. Avoidance, though, will help in *every* circumstance.

I hope I am proven wrong. For the sake of those suffering from food allergy, I hope there will one day be a magic pill that will eradicate food allergy forever and allow sufferers to eat what they wish!

Appendices

Appendices

Appendix A
Elimination Diets

Milk Elimination Diet

Milk is important to the diet because it contains calcium. However, eliminating calcium from your diet for three weeks poses no danger to your health. There is more than enough calcium stored in the body to last through the three-week diet, provided you have been ingesting adequate amounts of calcium before starting the diet.

Although eggs are considered a dairy product, they contain no milk. You may eat eggs during a milk elimination diet.

FOODS ELIMINATED	FOODS ALLOWED
All milk (including dried, evaporated, and skimmed), cream, yoghurt, and buttermilk	All meats, vegetables, and fruits
Cottage cheese and all other cheeses, pizza and other foods prepared with cheese, butter and most margarines	*Mocha Mix*, which is a locally obtainable cream substitute that can be purchased at food markets or health food stores. Use it on cereal and other foods, in coffee, and for cooking (pancakes and waffles). Some patients drink it after adding water, though nutritionally it is not a substitute for milk and does not contain calcium.
Ice cream and sherbert	
Creamed and mild soups, sauces and gravies, and mild puddings	

FOODS ELIMINATED	FOODS ALLOWED
Pancakes and waffles made with milk (most commercially-made mixes contain dried milk and should not be used)	*Soylac*, *Sobee*, and *Isomil*, which are soybean milks often substituted for cow's milk in the infant's diet and enjoyed by some older children. Can be substituted for milk in cooking (though it is sweeter in flavor than cow's milk). *Nutramigen* and *Gerber's* meat base are also substitutes for milk and may be purchased at most drug stores. For older children and adults on a general diet, no special substitute is required.
"Non-dairy" substitutes containing caseinate, such as *Coffeemate*, *Cereal Blend*, *Preem*, *Rich'ning*, *Imo*, *Cool Whip*, etc. Caseinate is a milk protein.	
Foods with whey, such as "imitation" milk and prepared mixes	Peach or pear juice or apricot nectar on dry cereal. A milk-free margarine such as *Nucoa* or *Willow Run* may be used on hot cereal. Stewed strawberries are excellent on dry cereal.
	Fruit ices (containing no milk, caseinate, or whey) are available at some stores— *read the label*. Popsicles and frozen fruit juices are also allowed. Keep a supply on hand in your freezer as a special treat when other children have ice cream.
	Hard candy, suckers, jelly beans, peanut brittle (without butter), gum drops, and licorice
	Root beer, *Squirt*, *Seven-Up*, orange, grape, and other carbonated or fruit drinks

Chocolate Elimination Diet

Chocolate is not important to the diet. This is impossible for some chocolate lovers to believe, but it's true. Eliminating chocolate from the diet poses no danger to your health.

FOODS ELIMINATED	FOODS ALLOWED
Chocolate candy, chocolate cookies and cake, chocolate pie, *Eskimo* pie, chocolate milk, chocolate flavorings, chocolate coated nuts Cocoa products Cola drinks, including diet colas like *Tab*. Cola drinks contain a chocolate product. Some dark rye breads, which may contain chocolate or cocoa	Most candies, suckers, jelly beans, peanut brittle, gum drops, licorice, and other chocolate-free candy. Carob (a chocolate substitute) is obtainable as a powder or candy bar at most health food stores. Though carob is free of chocolate, it is not superior nutritionally (as many people believe). Root beer, *Squirt*, *Seven-Up*, orange, grape, and other carbonated or fruit drinks

Salicylate Additive Elimination Diet

The salicylate additive group represents a family of substances that includes preservatives, artificial flavorings, coloring agents, and various chemicals. It can be confusing. Some additives contain salicylates, and some salicylates contain additives. You won't find the name "salicylate" on packages, and sometimes you don't find the word "additive" either. Instead, you must know whether additives or salicylates are in a food or you must learn clues that will tip you off. For additives, the clues are strange-sounding words like calcium-disodium, EDTA, BHA, sodium sulfite, sodium lauryl sulfate, and monosodium glutamate. For salicylates you may read "acetylsalicylic acid" or you may read nothing at all. Some natural foods like fruits contain salicylate. It may not make sense, but scientists provide us with this information. In cases where there is scientific disagreement about a food, you should avoid it to be sure you don't overlook any possibility. Remember—this is only for three weeks.

FOODS ELIMINATED

Almonds
Apples
Apricots
Blackberries
Cherries
Cucumbers and pickles
Currants
Gooseberries
Grapes and raisins
Nectarines
Oranges
Peaches
Plums and prunes
Raspberries
Strawberries
Tomatoes

Ice cream
Oleomargarine
Breakfast cereal with artificial
   flavor
Cake mixes
Bakery goods (except plain
   bread)
Gelatin products
Commercial candies
Chewing gum
Frankfurters
Cloves
Oil of Wintergreen
Toothpaste and toothpowder
Mint flavors

FOODS ALLOWED

All meats, except those that are artificially flavored, such as frankfurters, bologna, etc.

All fish, except fish sticks, fish patties, and fish cakes

Eggs

Milk and milk products

Butter (without food coloring added) or *Willow Run* margarine (purchased at a health food store)

All vegetables, except cucumbers and tomatoes

All starches, such as plain bread, rice, potatoes, pancake mixes (without coloring)

Fruit (grapefruit, lemons, pears, bananas, dates, limes, and figs)

Beverages (coffee and *Seven-Up*)

Pure maple syrup, all vegetable oils, distilled white vinegar, salt, and pepper

You may use *Tylenol* instead of aspirin for a fever or headache. This can be pur-

FOODS ELIMINATED	FOODS ALLOWED

FOODS ELIMINATED

Lozenges
Mouthwash
Jam or jelly
Lunch meats (salami,
  bologna, etc.)

Cider and cider vinegars
Wine and wine vinegars
Kool Aid and similar
  beverages
Soda pop (all soft drinks)
Diet drinks and supplements
Gin and all distilled drinks
  (except Vodka)
All tea
Beer

All medicines containing
aspirin, such as *Bufferin,
Anacin, Excedrin, Alka-Seltzer,
Empirin, Darvon Compound,
Coricidin, APC, Dristan,
4-Way*

Perfumes

*Anything containing artificial
color (sometimes called tar-
trazine), artificial flavors, or preservatives*

FOODS ALLOWED

chased at a pharmacy without a prescription.

Corn Elimination Diet

Traces of corn appear in a wide variety of foods because corn
is relatively inexpensive. The trial diet will not be worth doing
unless corn in *any* form is avoided. If there is any question
regarding a prepared food, check the ingredients listed on the
label. You should eliminate corn syrup, corn starch, and corn
meal.

FOODS ELIMINATED

All foods made with fresh corn, such as canned, frozen, or roasted corn, and grits

Foods that contain dried corn, such as corn flakes, corn meal, corn starch, and popcorn

All refined forms of corn, such as corn syrup, corn oil, corn sugars, dextrose, glucose, dextrin, fructose, maltodextrin, lactic acid

Hidden sources of corn are flours, sweetened fruits, ice cream, sherbert ice, processed or canned meats, containers for packaging of foods, canned or frozen vegetables.

Many medications and vitamins contain corn as a binder or sweetener.

Baking mixes, beers, breads, candy, ketchups, cereals, cookies, paper cups, processed fish, fried foods, fruit juices, ice creams, jams, margarines, milk in paper cartons, peanut butters, puddings, salad dressing, sausages, spaghetti, cream soups, syrups, vinegar, whiskies, wines, salt, powdered sugar, pickles, leavening agents and yeast, chewing gum, baby food, carbo-

FOODS ALLOWED

Cereals: *Kellogg's Rice Krispies, Nabisco's Shredded Wheat*

Coffee: *Instant Folgers*

Cookies: Certain *Pepperidge Farm* varieties

Soft Drinks: *Kool-Aid* (presweetened), *Saftway Cragmont Strawberry* or *Orange, Welchade Grape Juice*

Sweeteners: Maple syrup, honey, and sugar

Cooking Oil: Safflower

FOODS ELIMINATED

nated beverages, instant coffee, toothpaste

Remember to read labels. Home preparation is the key.

Wheat Elimination Diet

Traces of wheat occur in a wide variety of foods. Check the ingredients listed on the label.

FOODS ELIMINATED	FOODS ALLOWED
Baby foods, such as mixed cereal, cookies, teething biscuits, prepared puddings and custards	As a substitute for hot wheat cereal you may use cornmeal mush, oatmeal, or *Cream of Rice*.
Breads, cakes, cookies, crackers, pretzels	As a dry cereal you may use *Corn Flakes, Rice Krispies, Puffed Rice*, and rice flakes.
Breakfast foods that contain wheat, such as *Cream of Wheat, Pablum, Grapenuts, Farina, Ralston's Pep, Puffed Wheat, Shredded Wheat*, wheat germ, wheat starch, etc. *Use no bran.*	The *only* bread substitute easily purchased that you may use is *Ry-Krisp* crackers. If desired, rice cookies, rice bread, and wheat-free soy bean bread may be used.
Flour or flour products, such as macaroni, spaghetti noodles, vermicelli, ravioli, gluten flour, graham flour	Rice flour, cornstarch, potato starch, arrowroot, lima bean flour, or tapioca may be used to thicken soups, gravies, or sauces.
Pastry pies, bread crumbs, batters (waffles and pancakes), and cones	

FOODS ELIMINATED

Postum, *Ovaltine*, malted milk, certain canned soups, beer, ale

Sauces, chowders, soups, gravies, or *any* other food prepared with flour or containing noodles

Sausage, hamburger, meatloaf (unless ground at home without wheat filler) or croquettes, fish rolled in crackers, wiener schnitzel, chili con carne, or canned baked beans

This is a partial list. Read the labels.

Appendix B
Sample Menu Plan
From A Registered
Dietician

Menu Plan For A Milk, Corn
and Chocolate-Free Diet

Breakfast	Lunch	Dinner
1 cup orange juice	1 cup homemade	Green salad (with
1 egg	vegetable soup	vinegar and
2 strips bacon	Rice wafer	sesame or soy-
Sourdough French	3 oz. roast turkey	bean oil)
bread	1 cup steamed rice	3 oz. roast beef
(Read the label	1 serving vegetable	Large baked potato
for corn prod-	*Nucoa* margarine	*Nucoa* margarine
ucts. Many	Fresh fruit	2 servings vege-
breads have corn	Lemonade	tables
products added		Sourdough French
or are dusted		bread (check for
with corn prod-		corn products)
ucts.)		Gelatin with fresh
Margarine (*Nucoa*)		fruit
Cream of Wheat		Lemonade
(with *Nucoa* mar-		
garine and		
brown sugar)		
Soy milk		

This meal is approximately 1900–2000 calories.

Appendix C
Recipes For
Allergy-Free Cooking

This section contains recipes for the food-sensitive individual. You should not confuse a restricted diet with a bland, tasteless, or boring one. Hours of research have been devoted to devising meals that in many cases taste better than the original.

There are substitutes for eggs, chocolate, breads, cakes, cookies, main courses, and ice cream. The nutritional value of these substitutes and meals is often higher than the foods they replace. They are the kinds of meals that can be enjoyed by the entire family, thus eliminating the need to cook separately for the allergic individual.

The recipes are grouped together as Soups, Vegetables and Sauces, Main Courses, Breads and Muffins, and Desserts. This appendix is not meant as an encyclopedia of recipes. It is meant to show you the variety of possibilities. If you want additional recipes, you can find them in health food stores and libraries. Many individuals create their own recipes for those foods they miss the most.

In Canada there is an organization called the Allergy Information Association. It is composed of lay people who have joined together because of their common interest in allergy and their desire to share information. They publish a newsletter, and for a nominal fee anyone can join. Members receive the newsletter and can send in questions, which are answered by an advisory board. I recommend the Association highly. (See Appendix E for this and other useful addresses.)

SUBSTITUTIONS AND EQUIVALENTS

Before turning to the recipes, you should read the following general rules for making substitutions. You will see how these substitutes are implemented in the recipes, and with practice you can adapt your own recipes.

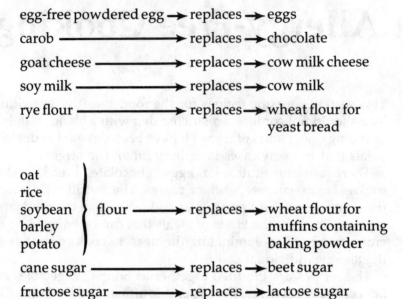

egg-free powdered egg → replaces → eggs

carob ⟶ replaces → chocolate

goat cheese ⟶ replaces → cow milk cheese

soy milk ⟶ replaces → cow milk

rye flour ⟶ replaces → wheat flour for yeast bread

oat
rice
soybean ⎬ flour ⟶ replaces → wheat flour for
barley   muffins containing
potato   baking powder

cane sugar ⟶ replaces → beet sugar

fructose sugar ⟶ replaces → lactose sugar

EQUIVALENTS AND GENERAL COMMENTS

Many of the wheat-free recipes contain higher than normal amounts of baking powder and eggs. This compensates for the absence of gluten, which holds the dough together.

The following is a table of equivalents for 1 cup of wheat flour.

1 cup of wheat flour   =   1½ cups rye flour
                             1 cup rye meal
                             1 cup corn flour
                             1 cup fine cornmeal
                             ¾ cup coarse cornmeal
                             ⅞ cup rice flour
                             1⅓ cups ground rolled oats
                             ⅝ cup potato flour
                             ½ cup barley flour

The following is the equivalent of 1 tablespoon of wheat flour when you are thickening sauces, gravies, or puddings.

1 tablespoon of wheat   =   1 tablespoon rice flour
  2 teaspoons instant tapioca
  ½ tablespoon arrowroot starch
  ½ tablespoon cornstarch
  ½ tablespoon potato
    starch flour

When you make cake mixes that require eggs, you can generally substitute 1 teaspoon of baking powder for each egg. Water can often be substituted for milk.

Soups

Cream Soup

Wheat- and Egg-Free, and no Milk

1 No. 2 can of vegetables*
1 tablespoon cornstarch
¼–½ teaspoon salt
1 cup *Isomil* (or other soy milk)
1 tablespoon vegetable shortening

Drain vegetables, reserving liquid. Press vegetables through coarse sieve and set aside. Pour 1½ cups vegetable liquid into 1-quart saucepan. If there is not enough vegetable liquid to make 1½ cups, add water to make up the difference. Sprinkle cornstarch and salt on surface of liquid and let stand for a few minutes; stir until cornstarch is blended in. Stir in *Isomil* (or other soy milk). Add shortening. Heat to a boil, stirring constantly, and then boil gently for 5 minutes. Stir in the sieved vegetable and reheat to serving temperature.

Makes 2½ cups.

* Use vegetables such as peas, green beans and carrots which are included in your diet. Two cups of fresh or frozen vegetables cooked in two cups of boiling water may be used in place of canned vegetables.

Cream Soup (Different Variety)

Corn- and Egg-Free, and no Milk

> 1 tablespoon vegetable shortening
> 1½ tablespoons flour
> ¼–½ teaspoon salt
> 1 cup *Isomil* (or other soy milk)
> 1 cup water
> 1 cup cooked, strained or mashed
>   vegetable*

Melt shortening in saucepan over low heat. Remove from heat and blend in the flour and salt. Gradually stir in the *Isomil* or other soy milk, keeping mixture smooth. Stir in the water. Cook over medium heat, stirring constantly, until thickened. Blend in vegetable; heat to serving temperature and serve at once.

Makes 3 cups.

* Use vegetables such as peas, spinach, asparagus, celery and potatoes which are included in your diet. Liquid drained from the cooked vegetable may be used in place of water to enhance the flavor and food value.

Tomato Cream Soup

Egg-, Wheat-, and Corn-Free, and no Milk

> 1¼ cups condensed tomato soup*
> ⅔ cup water
> ⅔ cup *Isomil* (or other soy milk)

Blend together all ingredients in a saucepan. Cook over low heat to serving temperature. Serve at once.

Makes 2½ cups.

* Canned condensed soups not containing milk or strained vegetables may be used in place of the condensed tomato soup.

Vegetables and Sauces

Medium White Sauce

No Wheat or Egg

>2 tablespoons *Nucoa* or *Mazola*
>   margarine
>1 tablespoon *Argo* cornstarch
>½ teaspoon salt
>⅛ teaspoon pepper
>1 cup milk

Melt margarine in saucepan. Stir in cornstarch, salt and pepper. Remove from heat. Gradually add milk, mixing until smooth. Bring to boil over medium heat, stirring constantly, and boil 1 minute.

Makes about 1 cup.

Almond Sauce: Stir 2 tablespoons toasted chopped blanched almonds into Medium White Sauce. Serve with fish or vegetables.

Cheese Sauce: Stir ¼ cup finely shredded cheese into Medium White Sauce, stirring until cheese is melted. Serve with vegetables or croquettes.

Creamed Dishes: Stir ½ to ¾ cup cooked diced meat, flaked fish or vegetables into Medium White Sauce.

Scalloped Dishes: Prepare double recipe Medium White Sauce. Mix in 1 to 1½ cups cooked meat, fish or vegetables. Pour into 1-quart casserole. Sprinkle with paprika. Bake in 375°F (moderate) oven 25 to 30 minutes or until thoroughly heated.

Cherry Sauce

No Wheat or Milk

> 1 (1-pound) can pitted sour red cherries
> 2 tablespoons *Argo* cornstarch
> Pinch cinnamon
> 1 cup *Karo* light corn syrup
> Red food coloring (optional)

Drain and reserve liquid from cherries adding water, if necessary, to make ⅔ cup. Combine cornstarch and cinnamon in
medium saucepan. Gradually stir in cherry liquid; add cherries.
Stir in light corn syrup. Stirring constantly, bring to a boil over
medium heat and boil for 1 minute. Add red food coloring, if
desired. Serve warm over sponge cake.

Makes 2½ cups.

White Sauce

Corn- and Egg-Free, and no Milk

> 1–2 tablespoons vegetable shortening*
> 1½–3 tablespoons flour
> ¼ teaspoon salt
> ½ cup *Isomil* (or other soy milk)
> ½ cup water

Melt shortening in saucepan over low heat. Remove from heat
and blend in flour and salt. Gradually stir in *Isomil* or other soy
milk, keeping mixture smooth. Stir in water. Cook over medium
heat, stirring constantly, until mixture thickens.

* First two ingredients will vary in the amount used, depending on how thick
you would like the consistency to be. A medium sauce may be used for
creamed and scalloped dishes of vegetables, meat, poultry or fish; a thick
sauce may be used to make croquettes.

Mashed Potatoes Deluxe

No Milk

> 1 medium-sized potato
> 1½ tablespoons diluted *Isomil* (or other
>   soy milk)
> Salt and pepper to taste

Scrub potato. Cook in boiling water until tender. Remove skin. Mash potato and season to taste with salt and pepper. Beat in diluted *Isomil* or other soy milk until potato is white and fluffy.

Makes 1 serving.

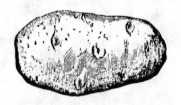

Zippy Potato Topping

No Wheat or Milk

> 1 cup *Hellmann's* or *Best Foods*
>   real mayonnaise
> 2 medium green onions, cut up
> 2 large pimiento-stuffed olives
> 1 small stalk celery, cut up
> 1 small clove garlic

Place real mayonnaise, green onions, olives, celery and garlic in blender container; cover. Blend until smooth. Cover, chill.

Makes about 1¾ cups.

Continental Lemon Sauce

No Wheat or Milk

    1 cup *Hellmann's* or *Best Foods*
      real mayonnaise
    2 eggs
    3 tablespoons lemon juice
    ½ teaspoon salt
    ½ teaspoon dry mustard

In small saucepan with wire whisk, beat together real mayonnaise, eggs, lemon juice, salt and dry mustard until smooth. Stirring constantly, cook over medium-low heat until thick (do not boil). Serve over vegetables, seafood or poached eggs.

Makes about 1⅔ cups.

Main Courses

Meat-Rice Patties

Egg- and Wheat-Free, and no Milk

    ½ pound ground beef
    ¾ cup cooked rice
    ½–¾ teaspoon salt
    ¼ cup *Isomil* (or other soy milk)

Combine all ingredients. Shape into patties, using ¼ cup mixture for each patty. Place on broiler pan, three inches from heat, and cook until browned; turn and heat until browned on other side. Serve hot.

Makes 6 patties.

Tuna-Potato Jubilee

Milk- and Egg-Free

> 2 cups boiled potatoes, sliced thin
> 1 tablespoon chopped parsley
> 1 7 oz. can tuna fish, drained
> 1 tablespoon diced onion
> 1 cup Medium White Sauce
> (see recipe earlier)
> Salt, pepper, paprika to taste

Preheat oven to 425°F. Arrange sliced potatoes in a greased, shallow, 1-quart casserole. Flake the tuna over the potatoes and sprinkle with onion, parsley, salt, pepper and paprika. Cover with the *Isomil* White Sauce and sprinkle top with additional paprika. Bake 25 minutes, or until bubbly and slightly browned on top.

Makes 6 servings.

Crepe Lasagne

No Wheat

> 1 container (15 oz.) ricotta cheese
> 1 egg, slightly beaten
> ½ cup grated Parmesan cheese
> 4 cups Meat Sauce (recipe follows)
> 6 Cornstarch Crepes (recipe below)
> 8 oz. mozzarella cheese, shredded

Stir together ricotta, egg and ¼ cup Parmesan. In deep 2-quart casserole, spread ¾ cup Meat Sauce. Top with 1 crepe, ⅓ cup ricotta mixture, ½ cup Meat Sauce and ⅓ cup mozzarella. Repeat with remaining ingredients. Sprinkle with Parmesan. Bake in 350°F oven 45 to 55 minutes or until bubbly. Let stand 20 minutes.

Makes 6 servings.

Meat Sauce: In 3-quart saucepan, heat 2 tablespoons *Mazola* corn oil over medium heat. Add 1 pound lean ground beef, ½ cup chopped onion, ¼ cup chopped parsley and 1 large clove garlic, minced. Stirring frequently, cook 10 minutes or until beef is browned. Place 1 can (28 oz.) tomatoes in blender container; cover. Blend on high 30 seconds or until finely chopped. Add to meat mixture. Stir in 1 can (6 oz.) tomato paste, 1 teaspoon sugar, 1 teaspoon dried basil leaves, ½ teaspoon salt, ½ teaspoon dried oregano leaves and ⅛ teaspoon pepper. Bring to boil. Reduce heat and simmer, stirring occasionally, 45 minutes.

Makes 4 cups.

Cornstarch Crepes

No Wheat

> 2 eggs
> ¾ cup milk
> 6 tablespoons *Argo* or *Kingsford's*
>   cornstarch
> 1 tablespoon *Mazola* corn oil
> ¾ teaspoon baking powder
> ⅛ teaspoon salt

Place all ingredients in blender container, cover. Blend on high speed 1 minute or until smooth. Pour about 2 tablespoons batter into center of hot, greased 6-inch crepe pan or skillet. Turn and twist immediately to cover bottom of pan. Cook about 30 seconds over medium-high heat until lightly browned and top dries around edge. Turn and cook on other side several seconds. Turn out onto waxed paper-lined tray. Repeat with remaining batter.

Makes 12 crepes.

Note: Unfilled crepes may be stored a few days in refrigerator between layers of waxed paper in a plastic bag. They may also be stored in freezer several weeks.

Crispy Chicken

No Wheat or Milk

> 3 cups crisp rice cereal,
>   finely crushed
> 1 teaspoon paprika
> ½ teaspoon salt
> ¼ teaspoon pepper
> 1 broiler-fryer chicken,
>   cut in parts
> ½ cup *Hellmann's* or *Best Foods*
>   real mayonnaise

Place first four ingredients in large plastic food bag; shake well. Brush chicken on all sides with real mayonnaise. Add to bag one piece at a time; shake to coat. Place on rack in broiler pan. Bake in 425°F oven 40 to 45 minutes or until golden brown and tender.

Makes 4 servings.

Ham Tostadas

No Wheat or Egg

> 1 can (15 to 16 oz.) pinto or
>   red kidney beans
> 4 tablespoons *Mazola* corn oil
> 4 (7") corn tortillas
> 2 cups shredded lettuce
> 4 oz. cooked ham, cut in strips
> 4 oz. Cheddar cheese, cut in strips
> Tostada Dressing (recipe follows)

In skillet, coarsely mash beans with bean liquid. Stir in 2 tablespoons corn oil. Stirring constantly, cook over medium heat 10 minutes or until all liquid is absorbed; set aside. In small skillet, heat remaining corn oil over medium heat. Add tortillas, one at a time. Fry, turning once, 1 to 2 minutes or until crisp. Drain on paper towels. Spread each tortilla generously with bean mixture. Top with ½ cup lettuce and strips of ham and cheese. Serve with Tostada Dressing.

Makes 4 servings.

Tostada Dressing: In jar with tight fitting lid, combine ⅔ cup *Mazola* corn oil, ⅓ cup wine vinegar, ½ teaspoon salt, ½ teaspoon brown sugar, ½ teaspoon paprika, ½ teaspoon dry mustard, ¼ teaspoon pepper and ⅛ teaspoon hot pepper sauce. Cover; shake well. Chill. Shake before serving.

Makes 1 cup.

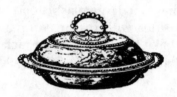

Saucy Meatballs

No Milk, Wheat or Egg

> 5 tablespoons *Argo* or *Kingsford's* cornstarch
> 2 cups homemade beef broth*
> ¼ cup chopped parsley
> ¼ teaspoon dried rosemary leaves, crushed
> ⅛ teaspoon pepper
> 1 pound ground beef
> 2 tablespoons *Mazola* corn oil
> 1 cup sliced mushrooms
> ⅓ cup sliced green onion
> ½ cup dry white wine
> Cooked rice

Stir together 2 tablespoons cornstarch, ¼ cup broth, parsley, rosemary and pepper. Add beef; mix well. Let stand 10 minutes. Shape into 20 meatballs. Roll in 2 tablespoons cornstarch. In large skillet, heat 1 tablespoon corn oil over medium heat. Add meatballs; brown on all sides. Remove. If necessary, add remaining corn oil. Add mushrooms and onion. Sauté 2 minutes. Add 1 cup broth, wine and meatballs. Bring to boil. Reduce heat; cover and simmer 15 minutes. Mix remaining 1 tablespoon cornstarch and ¾ cup broth until smooth. Stir into skillet. Stirring constantly, bring to boil over medium heat and boil 1 minute. Serve over rice.

Makes 4 servings.

* Canned beef broth may contain hydrolyzed vegetable protein, which is often derived from wheat.

Vichyssoise

No Milk

> 4 cups water
> 1 pound potatoes, peeled, diced
> 2 cups chopped onion
> 6 chicken-flavored bouillon cubes*
> ½ teaspoon salt
> ¼ teaspoon white pepper
> ½ cup *Hellmann's* or *Best Foods*
>   real mayonnaise
> Chopped chives

In 4-quart saucepan, bring first 6 ingredients to boil over high heat. Reduce heat to low. Cover and simmer 15 minutes or until potatoes are tender; cool. Place half at a time in blender container; cover. Blend until smooth. Pour into large bowl. Stir in real mayonnaise. Cover; chill overnight. Garnish with chives.

Makes about 4 cups.

* May contain hydrolyzed vegetable protein, which is often derived from wheat.

Breads and Muffins

Yeast (Basic White) Bread

No Milk

> 5–6 cups all-purpose flour
> 3 tablespoons sugar
> 2 teaspoons salt
> 2 packages active dry yeast
> 1½ cups water
> ¼ cup vegetable oil or shortening
> ½ cup *Isomil Concentrated Liquid*
>   (*Do not use Isomil Ready To Feed*)

In a large mixing bowl combine 2 cups flour, sugar, salt and yeast. Blend well. In small saucepan, heat water and oil or shortening until very warm (120°F to 130°F). Add warm liquid and *Isomil Concentrated Liquid* to flour mixture. Blend at low speed until moistened; beat 3 minutes at medium speed. Stir in additional flour (2½ to 3 cups) until dough clings to dough hook and cleans sides of bowl. Knead on medium speed for 7 to 10 minutes longer or until dough is smooth and elastic. Dough will be slightly sticky to the touch. Place dough in greased bowl, turning to grease top. Cover loosely with plastic wrap and cloth. Let rise in warm place until light and doubled in size, about 1½ hours. Punch down several times to remove all air bubbles. Let dough rest for 15 minutes. Divide dough in half and roll each half into a rectangle, approximately 9″ x 14″. A rolling pin will smooth dough and remove gas bubbles. Starting at short end, roll dough tightly. Pinch dough to seal ends. Place, seam side down in a 9″ × 5″ × 3″ greased loaf pan. Cover; let rise in warm place free from drafts, until doubled in bulk, about 1 hour. Bake in preheated 400°F oven for 25 to 30 minutes *or* until nicely browned. When loaves are done, they will sound hollow when rapped with the knuckles. Remove bread from pans immediately; cool on racks before slicing. If a soft crust is desired, brush tops of loaves with melted margarine.

Makes 2 loaves, 18 slices per loaf.

Quick Pecan Muffins

No Wheat

        3 cups *H-O Instant Oatmeal*
        ⅓ cup firmly packed brown sugar
        3¼ teaspoons baking powder
        1 teaspoon salt
        ½ cup coarsely chopped pecans
        ½ cup chopped dates or raisins
        ⅓ cup *Nucoa* or *Mazola* margarine
        1 cup milk
        2 eggs, beaten

Grease 12 (2½"·× 1¼") muffin pans. Toss oatmeal, brown sugar, baking powder and salt together in mixing bowl. Stir in nuts and fruit. Melt margarine. Remove from heat; stir in milk. Add eggs; beat until well blended. Add all at once to oatmeal mixture. Mix well. Pour into muffin pans. Bake in 425°F (hot) oven about 25 minutes or until muffins test done.

Makes 12.

Date and Nut Muffins

No Egg or Milk

        ¾ teaspoon baking soda
        1 (8 oz.) package pitted dates,
          chopped
        ¾ cup boiling water
        ¼ cup *Mazola* corn oil
        1½ cups sifted flour
        ½ cup sugar
        ¼ cup chopped nuts
        ½ teaspoon vanilla

Grease 12 (2½″ × 1¼″) muffin pans. Sprinkle baking soda over dates in mixing bowl. Add boiling water and corn oil. Mix flour, sugar, and nuts together; add to date mixture. Add vanilla. Stir just until dry ingredients are moistened. Pour into prepared muffin pans, filling cups two-thirds full. Bake in 375°F (moderate) oven about 25 minutes or until muffins test done.

Makes 12 muffins.

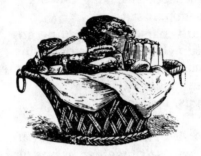

Corn Bread

No Wheat

> 2 cups yellow corn meal
> 2 tablespoons sugar
> 1½ teaspoons baking powder
> 1 teaspoon salt
> 2 eggs, beaten
> 1 cup milk
> ¼ cup *Mazola* corn oil

Grease 8″ × 8″ × 2″ baking pan. In medium bowl, stir together first 4 ingredients. In small bowl, stir together remaining ingredients. Stir into corn meal mixture just until moistened. Turn into pan. Bake in 400°F oven 20 to 25 minutes.

Makes 9 servings.

Jalapeño Corn Bread: Follow recipe for Corn Bread. Fold in 1 can (12 oz.) mexicorn, well drained, and 1 can (4 oz.) chopped green chilies, well drained. Top with ½ cup shredded Cheddar cheese.

Desserts

Caramel Custard

No Wheat

      4 teaspoons *Karo* dark corn syrup
      ¼ cup sugar
      3 tablespoons *Argo* cornstarch
      ⅛ teaspoon salt
      2 cups milk
      1 egg, well beaten
      1 teaspoon vanilla

Pour 1 teaspoon corn syrup into each of 4 custard cups, swirling cup to coat sides. Mix sugar, cornstarch and salt in double boiler top. Gradually stir in milk. Cook over boiling water, stirring constantly until mixture thickens. Cover; cook 10 minutes longer. Remove from boiling water; blend a little mixture into egg, then stir into hot mixture. Cook over boiling water 2 minutes, stirring constantly. Remove from heat; stir in vanilla. Pour into custard cups. Chill. Unmold to serve.

Makes 4 servings.

Lemon-Orange Sherbet

No Wheat, Egg, or Milk

      3 cups water
      1 cup *Karo* light corn syrup
      ¾ cup sugar
      1 tablespoon grated lemon rind
      1 envelope unflavored gelatin
      ⅔ cup lemon juice
      ½ cup orange juice

Mix together water, corn syrup, sugar and lemon rind in 3-quart saucepan. Cook over medium heat, stirring constantly, until sugar is dissolved and mixture comes to boil. Boil 5 minutes. Remove from heat. Meanwhile, sprinkle gelatin over lemon juice to soften. Add to hot mixture and stir until gelatin is dissolved. Add orange juice. Cool to lukewarm. If desired, strain. Pour into 9 " × 5 " × 3" loaf pan and freeze 3 to 4 hours or until mixture is firm. Turn into large chilled bowl. Wash and dry pan to prevent icy layer from forming on bottom. Beat until smooth and fluffy but not melted. Return to loaf pan. Freeze about 3½ hours or until firm.

Makes 14 (½ cup) servings.

Ginger Pear Dessert

No Wheat, Egg, or Milk

> 1 (1 pound, 13 oz.) can pear halves
> 1½ tablespoons *Argo* cornstarch
> ¼ cup slivered candied ginger or
>   ¼ teaspoon ground ginger
> ½ teaspoon grated lemon rind
> Currant jelly

Drain pears and reserve syrup. Mix cornstarch and reserved pear syrup in 2-quart saucepan. Add ginger and lemon rind. Heat over medium heat, stirring constantly, until mixture comes to a boil and boils 1 minute. Add pears, reduce heat and simmer 2 to 3 minutes. Arrange pears in serving dish, cut side up. Fill center of each pear with currant jelly. Pour syrup mixture over pears. Serve warm or chilled.

Makes 3 to 4 servings.

Baked Apples

No Wheat, Egg, or Milk

>6 medium baking apples
>¼ cup *Skippy* creamy or chunk style
>   peanut butter
>1 cup *Karo* light or dark corn syrup
>½ cup water
>½ teaspoon cinnamon

Core apples; peel upper half. Place in shallow baking dish. Stir peanut butter and ¼ cup corn syrup together until blended; spoon into centers of apples. Mix remaining ¾ cup corn syrup with water and cinnamon. Pour over apples. Bake in 350°F (moderate) oven, basting frequently, about 1 hour or until apples are tender. Serve hot or cold.

Makes 6 servings.

Old-Fashioned Ice Cream

No Milk

>4 cans *Isomil* (or other soy milk)
>½ cup clear corn syrup
>2 packets (1 tablespoon/packet)
>   unflavored gelatin—soften in
>½ cup cold water
>1 cup sugar—add to gelatin and heat
>   slowly to dissolve sugar and gelatin;
>   cool
>¼ cup salad/cooking oil
>7 teaspoons vanilla extract

Mix all ingredients* and freeze in a one-gallon or 5-quart ice cream freezer. After the mix is frozen, remove and store in freezing compartment of refrigerator.

* Individual flavor variations: any fruits you like which are included in your diet may be added to recipe prior to freezing after being mashed or pureed in a blender.

Magnolia White Layer Cake

No Milk

⅔ cup all-vegetable margarine
3 cups sifted cake flour (sift before
    measuring)
½ cup *Isomil* (or other soy milk)
½ cup water
1½ cups sugar
3 eggs
4½ teaspoons baking powder
½ teaspoon salt
1 teaspoon vanilla

Preheat oven to 350°F. Grease and lightly flour two 8-inch round cake pans. Combine margarine and sugar in mixing bowl and cream until light and fluffy. Add eggs one at a time, beating well after each addition. Combine dry ingredients. Combine liquid ingredients. Add dry and wet ingredients alternately to mixing bowl, blending until smooth after each addition. Pour into prepared pans. Bake 40–45 minutes or until done. Cook 5 minutes in pan. Remove from pan and cool completely on cake rack.

Makes 2 layers.

Rich Chocolate Fudge

No Milk

> 2 cups sugar
> ¼ cup corn syrup
> ¼ cup water
> 2 tablespoons margarine
> 2 tablespoons cocoa
> ¼ cup *Isomil* (or other soy milk)
> 1 teaspoon vanilla

Mix sugar, cocoa and corn syrup in large saucepan. Add *Isomil* or other soy milk and water and mix until smooth. Cook over moderate heat, stirring until a soft ball forms in cold water (230°F on candy thermometer). Remove from heat and add margarine and vanilla. Beat until fudge starts to turn dull. Then pour into greased pan. Let stand until hardened; cut into 1-inch squares.

Buttercream Frosting

No Milk

> 1 pound powdered sugar
> ⅓ teaspoon salt
> 3–4 tablespoons *Isomil* (or other
>   soy milk)
> ½ cup margarine
> 1 teaspoon vanilla

Cream ⅓ sugar with margarine and salt in large bowl. Blend in vanilla and 2 tablespoons *Isomil* or other soy milk. Add remaining sugar to mixture. Gradually stir in remaining *Isomil* or other soy milk until desired spreading consistency is reached.

Frosts 2 layers.

Indian Pudding

Wheat- and Egg-Free, and no Milk

> ¼ cup yellow cornmeal
> ¼ cup water
> 1 cup *Isomil* (or other soy milk)
> 1 cup boiling water
> ½ cup raisins or finely cut prunes
> ½ cup molasses

Combine cornmeal and the ¼ cup water in top of double boiler. Let stand for 5 minutes. Stir in *Isomil* or other soy milk and then the boiling water. Cook over boiling water, stirring often, until thickened, about 20 minutes. Mix in raisins or chopped prunes and molasses. Pour into greased 1-quart casserole or baking dish. Bake in a slow oven (325°F) for 2 hours. Serve hot.

Makes 4–6 servings.

Macaroons

No Wheat or Milk

> 1¼ cups ground blanched almonds
> ¾ cup sugar
> 2 unbeaten egg whites
> 2 tablespoons *Argo* or *Kingsford's*
>   cornstarch
> 2 teaspoons water
> ¼ teaspoon vanilla
> 18 to 20 blanched almond halves

In bowl, mix ground almonds and sugar. Add egg whites, reserving about 1 tablespoon to brush on top of macaroons. Stir until well blended. Add next 3 ingredients, stirring well after each addition. Drop batter onto foil-covered baking sheet by teaspoonfuls 3 inches apart. Brush cookies with remaining egg white, then place almond half on top of each. Bake in 375°F oven 15 minutes or until evenly browned. Cool on wire rack 3 to 4 minutes or until foil can be peeled off. Remove foil; cool on rack.

Makes about 1½ dozen.

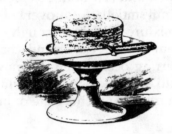

Crunchy Chews

No Wheat, Milk, or Egg

> ¾ cup sugar
> ¾ cup *Karo* light or dark corn syrup
> ¾ cup *Skippy* super chunk peanut butter
> 4½ cups corn flakes
> ¾ cup peanuts (optional)

Line 13″ × 9″ × 2″ baking pan with greased foil. In saucepan, mix sugar and corn syrup. Stirring constantly, bring to boil over medium heat. Boil 1 minute. Stir in peanut butter. Mix in corn flakes and nuts. Turn into pan. Press together firmly. Cool. Remove from pan. Cut into 1¹/₂ inch squares.

Makes about 4½ dozen.

Blanc Mange

No Wheat or Egg

½ cup sugar
5 tablespoons *Argo* cornstarch
¼ teaspoon salt
4 cups milk
1½ teaspoons vanilla

Mix sugar, cornstarch and salt in double boiler top. Gradually add milk, stirring until smooth. Cook over boiling water, stirring constantly, until mixture thickens enough to mound slightly when dropped from spoon. Cover and continue cooking 10 minutes longer, stirring occasionally. Remove from heat. Stir in vanilla. Pour into serving dish or individual dishes. Chill. Serve plain or with fresh fruit, chocolate or butterscotch sauce, jelly or jam.

Makes 6 to 8 servings.

Glazed Fresh Strawberry Pie

No Egg or Milk

1 baked (9-inch) pastry shell
3 pints strawberries, washed and
    hulled
1¼ cups sugar
3½ tablespoons *Argo* cornstarch
½ cup water
Few drops red food coloring

Mash 1 pint berries. Combine sugar and cornstarch in saucepan. Add water and mashed berries. Bring to boil over medium heat, stirring constantly, and boil 2 minutes. Remove from heat. Stir in food coloring. Cool. Fold remaining 2 pints berries into cooled mixture. Pile into pie shell. Chill.

Makes 6 to 8 servings.

All-Purpose Cookie

No Egg

> ½ cup *Argo* cornstarch
> ½ cup confectioners sugar
> 1 cup sifted flour
> ¾ cup *Nucoa* or *Mazola* margarine

Sift cornstarch, confectioners sugar and flour together into mixing bowl. Stir in margarine with spoon, mixing until soft dough forms. Prepare desired cookie variety as directed below. Bake in 300°F (slow) oven about 20 minutes or until edges are lightly browned.

Makes 2½ dozen.

Melting Moments: Shape All-Purpose Cookie dough into 1-inch balls. Place about 1½ inches apart on ungreased baking sheet; flatten with floured fork. Bake.

Jelly Center Cookies: Shape All-Purpose Cookie dough into 1-inch balls. Place about 1½ inches apart on ungreased baking sheet. Make an indentation in center of each ball. Bake. Fill indentations with jelly. For variety, roll dough balls in finely chopped nuts before placing on baking sheet.

Crescents: Mix ¼ cup finely chopped nuts into All-Purpose Cookie dough. Shape dough into rolls ½-inch thick and 3 inches long. Place on ungreased baking sheet, bending each roll into crescent shape. Bake.

Note: If dough is too soft to handle, cover and chill in refrigerator about 1 hour.

Oat Cookies

No Egg

       ½ cup sifted flour
       ½ teaspoon baking soda
       ½ teaspoon salt
       1½ cups *H-O Old-Fashioned Oats*
       ½ cup semi-sweet chocolate chips or
          chopped dried figs, raisins or dates
       ½ cup *Nucoa* or *Mazola* margarine
       ½ cup *Karo* dark corn syrup

Sift flour, baking soda and salt together into bowl. Stir in oats. Add chocolate or fruit. Stir together margarine and corn syrup in mixing bowl. Stir in oat mixture. Drop batter onto greased baking sheet by teaspoonfuls, 2 inches apart. Bake in 375°F (moderate) oven 10 to 12 minutes or until delicately browned. Let stand 2 minutes before removing from baking sheet.

Makes 2½ dozen.

Wheat-Free Cupcakes

No Wheat

       1 cup sifted *Argo* cornstarch
       1 teaspoon baking powder
       ⅓ cup *Nucoa* or *Mazola* margarine
       ⅓ cup sugar
       1 egg
       ¼ teaspoon vanilla
       3 tablespoons milk

Grease 8 (2½" × 1¼ ") cupcake pans. Sift together cornstarch and baking powder. Stir margarine and sugar until blended in small mixing bowl. Beat in egg and vanilla. Add cornstarch mixture alternately with milk; mix just until smooth after each addition. Turn into prepared cupcake pans, filling two-thirds full. Bake in 375°F (moderate) oven 12 to 15 minutes or until cupcakes test done. Serve with whipped cream and fruit.

Makes 8.

Pineapple Upside Down Cake

Wheat- and Egg-Free, and no Milk

> ¼ cup vegetable shortening
> ½ cup brown sugar, firmly packed
> 1½ cups sifted rye flour
> ½ cup *Isomil* (or other soy milk)
> ¾ cup sugar
> ¼ cup cornstarch
> 3 teaspoons baking powder
> ½–¾ teaspoon salt
> ½ cup water
> 1½ cups (No. 2 can) crushed pineapple,
>   well drained

Melt ¼ cup of the shortening in 9-inch square layer cake pan over low heat. Add brown sugar and stir until it melts. Spread mixture evenly in bottom of pan and remove pan at once from heat. Arrange pineapple evenly on sugar mixture and then set aside. Meanwhile, cream the remaining ¼ cup shortening until fluffy. Gradually beat in sugar and then continue beating until fluffy. Combine rye flour, cornstarch, baking powder and salt; sift. Combine *Isomil* or other soy milk and water. Divide flour mixture into three parts; divide *Isomil* or other soy milk into two parts. Add flour and the *Isomil* or other soy milk portions alternately to the sugar mixture, starting and ending with the flour mixture. Blend well after each addition. Turn batter into pan and spread evenly over pineapple. Bake in moderate oven (350°F) until the top center springs back when lightly touched with finger, about 45 to 50 minutes. Put cake pan upside down on serving plate and let stand a few minutes before removing pan. Serve cake hot or cold.

Makes a 9-inch cake.

Appendix D
Families of
Related Foods

In many cases, people who are allergic to one member of a family of foods will be allergic to other members of the same family. For example, those allergic to shrimp are often allergic to crabs and lobster. Those allergic to peanuts are often allergic to other members of the legume family, such as peas and beans.

This rule is not uniformly true, however, and people can sometimes tolerate members of the same family (especially if they limit their intake or decrease the frequency at which they eat the offending food by rotating the food in their diet).

The following pages list the commonly recognized groups of foods that you may encounter. It should be used as a basis for suspecting foods that are in the same family as foods that you know affect you. The technique of elimination that you learned in this book will provide you with the answer that is right for *you*.

No matter what is written, the proof of food allergy is in eating a food and experiencing a reaction. If your body tells you something different from the list, listen to your body.

There are dashes between groups of fish when the relationship between a particular fish and the ones above and below it are not 100% certain. This classification is based on that of Dr. Vaughn's *Biologic Classification of Foods*.

Animal Foods

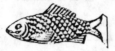

AMPHIBIANS
Frog

BIRDS
Chicken
  Chicken eggs
Duck
  Duck eggs
Goose
  Goose eggs
Turkey
Guinea hen
Squab
Pheasant
Partridge
Grouse

CRUSTACEANS
Crab
Crayfish
———
Lobster
———
Shrimp
———
Squid

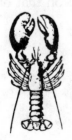

FISH
Sunfish
Bass
Perch
Snapper
Croaker
Weakfish
Drum
Scup
Porgy
———
Flounder
Sole
Halibut
———
Rosefish
———
Codfish
Scrod
Haddock
Hake
Pollack
Cusk
———
Sturgeon
Caviar
———
Anchovy
Sardine
Herring
Smelt

———
Trout
Salmon
Whitefish
Chub
Shad
———
Eel
———
Carp
Sucker
Buffalo
———
Catfish
Bullhead

———
Pike
Pickerel
Muskellunge
———
Mullet
Barracuda
———
Mackerel
Tuna
Pompano
Bluefish
Butterfish
Harvestfish
Swordfish

MAMMALS
Beef
  Veal
  Cow's milk
  Butter
  Cheese
  Gelatin
Pork
  Ham
  Bacon
Goat
  Goat's milk
  Cheese

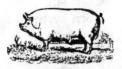

Mutton
  Lamb
Venison
Horse meat
Rabbit
Squirrel

MOLLUSKS
Abalone

———

Mussel
Oyster
Scallop
Clam

REPTILES
Turtle

Plant Foods

APPLE FAMILY
Apple
  Cider
  Vinegar
  Apple pectin
Pear
Quince
  Quince seed

ARROWROOT
  FAMILY
Arrowroot

ARUM FAMILY
Taro
  Poi

BANANA FAMILY
Banana

BEECH FAMILY
Chestnut

BIRCH FAMILY
Filbert
Hazelnut
Oil of birch
  (wintergreen)

BUCKWHEAT
  FAMILY
Buckwheat
Rhubarb

CASHEW FAMILY
Cashew
Pistachio
Mango

CITRUS FAMILY
Orange
Grapefruit
Lemon
Lime

Tangerine
Kumquat

COMPOSITE
  FAMILY
Leaf lettuce
Head lettuce
Endive
Escarole
Artichoke
Dandelion
Oyster plant
Chicory

EBONY FAMILY
Persimmon

FUNGI
Mushroom
Yeast

GINGER FAMILY
Ginger
Tumeric
Cardamon

GOOSEBERRY
   FAMILY
Gooseberry
Currant

GOOSEFOOT
   FAMILY
Beet
   Beet sugar
Spinach
Swiss chard

GOURD FAMILY
Pumpkin
Squash
Cucumber
Cantaloupe
Muskmelon
Honeydew melon
Persian melon
Casaba
Watermelon

GRAINS
Wheat
   Graham flour
   Gluten flour
   Bran
   Wheat germ
Oats
Rye
Barley
   Malt
Corn
   Cornstarch

Corn oil
Corn sugar
Corn syrup
Cerulose
Dextrose
Glucose
Rice
Wild rice
Sorghum
Cane
   Cane sugar
   Molasses

GRAPE FAMILY
Grape
   Raisin
   Cream of tartar

HEATH FAMILY
Cranberry
Blueberry

HONEYSUCKLE
   FAMILY
Elderberry

LAUREL FAMILY
Avocado
Cinnamon
Bay leaves

LECYTHIS
   FAMILY
Brazil nut

LEGUMES
Navy bean
Kidney bean

Lima bean
String bean
Soy bean
   Soy bean oil
Lentil
Black-eyed peas
Pea
Peanut
   Peanut oil
Licorice
Acacia
Senna

LILY FAMILY
Asparagus
Onion
Garlic
Leek
Chive
Aloes

MADDER FAMILY
Coffee

MALLOW
   FAMILY
Okra (Gumbo)
Cottonseed

MAPLE FAMILY
Maple syrup
   Maple sugar

MINT FAMILY
Mint
Peppermint
Spearmint
Thyme
Sage

Marjoram
Savory

MORNING
  GLORY
  FAMILY
Sweet potato
Yam

MULBERRY
  FAMILY
Mulberry
Fig
Hop
Breadfruit

MUSTARD
  FAMILY
Mustard
Cabbage
Cauliflower
Broccoli
Brussels sprouts
Turnip
Rutabaga
Kale
Collard
Celery cabbage
Kohlrabi
Radish
Horseradish
Watercress

MYRTLE FAMILY
Allspice
Cloves
Pimento
Paprika
Guava

NUTMEG FAMILY
Nutmeg

OLIVE FAMILY
Green olive
Ripe olive
  Olive oil

ORCHID FAMILY
Vanilla

PALM FAMILY
Coconut
Date
Sago

PAPAW FAMILY
Papaya

PARSLEY FAMILY
Parsley
Parsnip
Carrot
Celery
Celeriac
Caraway
Anise
Dill
Coriander
Fennel

PEDALIUM
  FAMILY
Sesame oil

PEPPER FAMILY
Black pepper

PINE FAMILY
Juniper

PINEAPPLE
  FAMILY
Pineapple

PLUM FAMILY
Plum
  Prune
Cherry
Peach
Apricot
Nectarine
Almond

POMEGRANATE
  FAMILY
Pomegranate

POPPY FAMILY
Poppy seed

POTATO FAMILY
Potato
Tomato
Eggplant
Red pepper
  Cayenne
Green pepper
Chili

ROSE FAMILY
Raspberry
Blackberry
Loganberry
Youngberry
Dewberry
Strawberry

SPURGE FAMILY
Tapioca

**STERCULA
  FAMILY**
Cocoa
  Chocolate

**SUNFLOWER
  FAMILY**
Jerusalem
  artichoke
Sunflower seed oil

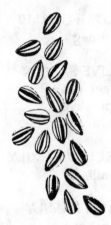

TEA FAMILY
Tea

WALNUT FAMILY
English walnut
Black walnut
Butternut
Hickory nut
Pecan

MISCELLANEOUS
Honey

Appendix E
Useful Addresses

Your Own Doctor

_____

_____

_____

Your Registered Dietician

_____

_____

_____

Your Allergist

_____

_____

_____

The Allergy Information
   Association
65 Tromley Drive
Islington, Ontario
Canada M9B 5Y7

The American Board of
   Allergy and Immunology
University City Science
   Center
3624 Market St.
Philadelphia, PA 19104

Center for Consumer Affairs
National Institute of Allergy
   and Infectious Disease
Office of Research Reporting
   and Public Response
9000 Rockville Pike
Bethesda, MD 20205

American Dietetic
   Association
430 North Michigan Ave.
Chicago, IL 60611

Appendix F
Lactase Deficiency and Milk Allergy

Many individuals experience watery diarrhea, nausea, bloating of the stomach, or cramping abdominal pain after eating milk products. They may think they are allergic to milk, but in fact they lack the enzyme that digests milk sugar. Their inability to digest the sugar causes fermentation in the gastrointestinal tract, production of gas, and the accumulation of water in the bowel. The gas and water are responsible for the symptoms.

This illness is known as lactase deficiency. Its symptoms are similar to the symptoms that true milk allergy can provoke. Lactase is the enzyme that digests the sugar lactose. Lactose is the sugar found in milk and milk products.

The deficiency of lactase may be partial or complete. This accounts for the variable severity. Those with total absence of lactase will have symptoms after ingesting small amounts of milk, while those with partial deficiency can tolerate substantial amounts of milk.

If you have been told you are allergic to milk and have only gastrointestinal symptoms, you should ask your doctor to test you for this condition. Patients who have been told they have dyspepsia, heartburn, and even ulcers may actually have this condition.

Treatment is identical to the treatment of milk allergy. *Avoid milk and milk-containing products.*

If you have total deficiency of the enzyme, you must avoid *all* milk products. If you have a partial deficiency, you must reduce your intake of lactose to a point you can tolerate. If you have a temporary deficiency, such as can occur during bowel infections, you need only be careful while you have the infection.

There are commercially-available milk substitutes for lactase deficiency. These products have predigested lactose or substitute sugars for lactose. Consult your doctor or registered dietician for the latest brands.

Appendix G
U.S. Food
Manufacturers

Below is a list of major U.S. food manufacturers, along with addresses and telephone numbers. If you find you have an allergic reaction to a particular product and are unable to pinpoint the specific ingredient provoking this response, you might want to contact them for further ingredient information.

Company/Division	Address/Phone #
The All American Gourmet Co.	One City Boulevard West #308 Orange, CA 92665 714/978-0772
American Home Foods	685 Third Avenue New York, NY 10017 212/878-5242
Amstar Corp.	1251 Avenue of the Americas New York, NY 10020 212/489-9000
Anderson Clayton Foods	WLCRC 3333 N. Central Expressway Richardson, TX 75080 214/231-6121

Company/Division	Address/Phone #
Armour Processed Meat Co.	15101 N. Scottsdale Road Scottsdale, AZ 85260 602/998-6282
Beatrice Meats, Inc.	1919 Swift Drive Oak Brook, IL 60522 312/850-5957
Beech-Nut Nutrition Corp.	P.O. Box 127 Fort Washington, PA 19034 215/628-9900
C & H Sugar Co.	1 California Street San Francisco, CA 94111 415/772-3869
Cadbury Schweppes, Inc.	6546 Pound Road Williamson, NY 14589 315/589-9613
Calif. Almond Growers Exchange (Blue Diamond)	P.O. Box 1768 Sacramento, CA 95808 916/446-8536 or 442-0771
Campbell Soup Co.	1 Campbell Place Camden, NJ 08101 609/342-3828 609/342-6022 609-342-4800
Carnation Company	5045 Wilshire Boulevard Los Angeles, CA 90036 213/932-6353
Chesebrough-Pond's, Inc.	40 Merritt Boulevard Trumbull, CT 06611 203/381-5529

Company/Division	Address/Phone #
The Clorox Co.	P.O. Box 24305 Oakland, CA 94623 415/271-7283
Coca-Cola USA	P.O. Drawer 1734 Atlanta, GA 30301 404/676-3228
Comstock Foods	P.O. Box 670 Rochester, NY 14602 716/385-6580
ConAgra Consumer Frozen Food Co.	P.O. Box 70 St. Louis, MO 63011 314/957-4073
Del Monte USA	P.O. Box 3575 San Francisco, CA 94119 415/442-4801 or 4802
Dole Food Co.	P.O. Box 7330 San Francisco, CA 94120 415/986-3000 ext. 4621
Dow Consumer Products, Inc.	9550 Zionsville Road Indianapolis, IN 46268 317/873-7093
Faultless Starch/ Bon Ami Co.	1025 W. 8th Street Kansas City, MO 64101 816/421-7075
Frito-Lay, Inc.	P.O. Box 660634 Dallas, TX 75266-0634 214/353-2112
General Foods Corp.	250 North Street White Plains, NY 10625 914/335-2500

Company/Division	Address/Phone #
General Mills, Inc.	P.O. Box 1113 Minneapolis, MN 55440 612/540-3201
Gerber Products Co.	445 State Street Fremont, MI 49412 616/928-2461
The Gorton Group	P.O. Box 361 Gloucester, MA 01930 617/283-3000 ext. 165
Heinz, USA	1062 Progress Street Pittsburgh, PA 15212 412/237-5695
Hershey Foods Corp.	P.O. Box 805 Hershey, PA 17033-0805 717/534-5130
Hillshire Farm Co.	P.O. Box 227 New London, WI 54961 414/982-2611
Hollywood Brands, Inc.	100 S. Poplar Centralia, IL 62804 618/532-4767
Interbake Foods, Inc.	P.O. Box 27487 Richmond, VA 23261 804/257-7454
International Multifoods	9449 Science Center Drive New Hope, MN 55428 612/340-3849
S. C. Johnson & Son	1525 Howe Street Racine, WI 53403 414/631-2427

Company/Division	Address/Phone #
Kellogg Co.	235 Porter Street P.O. Box 3423 Battle Creek, MI 49016-3423 616/961-2986 (VH) 616/961-2284 (RH) 616/961-3169 (VF)
Kraft, Inc.	R & D, 801 Waukegan Road Glenview, IL 60025 312/998-3576 312/998-2057 312/998-2054 312/998-4379
Land O'Lakes, Inc.	P.O. Box 116 Minneapolis, MN 55440-0016 612/481-2279
Lehn & Fink Products Group	225 Summit Avenue Montvale, NJ 07645 201/573-5788
Lever Brothers Co.	45 River Road Edgewater, NJ 07020 201/943-7100
Thomas J. Lipton, Inc.	800 Sylvan Avenue Englewood Cliffs, NJ 07632 201/894-7750
Malt-O-Meal Company	319 S. Water Street Northfield, MN 55057 612/645-6681
McCormick & Company, Inc.	414 Light Street Baltimore, MD 21202 301/547-6271

Company/Division	Address/Phone #
Minnetonka, Inc.	Jonathon Industrial Center Chaska, MN 55318 612/448-4181
Nabisco Brands, Inc.	500 Lanidex Plaza Parsippany, NJ 07054 201/428-5543
Nalley's Fine Foods	P.O. Box 11046 Tacoma, WA 98411 206/383-1621
National Oats Company, Inc.	1515 H Avenue, N.E. Cedar Rapids, IA 52402 319/364-9161
Nestlé Foods Corp.	100 Bloomingdale Road White Plains, NY 10605 914/682-6762
The NutraSweet Company	4711 Golf Road Skokie, IL 60076 312/982-7182
Ocean Spray Cranberries, Inc.	225 Water Street Plymouth, MA 02360 617/747-1000 ext. 246
The Old Fashioned Kitchen	1045 Towbin Avenue Lakewood, NJ 08701 201/364-4100
Ore-Ida Foods	P.O. Box 10 Boise, ID 83707 208/383-6237
Mrs. Paul's Kitchens	5501 Tabor Road Philadelphia, PA 19120 215/535-1151

Company/Division	Address/Phone #
Pepsi-Cola USA	Anderson Hill Road White Plains, NY 914/253-3295
Pepsico, Inc.	100 Stevens Avenue Valhalla, NY 10595 914/742-4505
The Pillsbury Company	Pillsbury Center M.S. 2818 200 S. 6th Street Minneapolis, MN 55402 612/330-8734
The Quaker Oats Company	617 W. Main Street Barrington, IL 60010 312/381-1980 ext. 2065 312/381-1980 ext. 2063
Ralston-Purina Company	Checkerboard Square St. Louis, MO 63164 314/982-2250
Reynolds Metals Company	6601 W. Broad Street Richmond, VA 23261 804/281-2109
Ross Laboratories	625 Cleveland Avenue Columbus, OH 43216 614/227-3333
Sandoz Nutrition	5320 W. 23rd Street P.O. Box 370 Minneapolis, MN 55440 612/925-6553
Kitchens of Sara Lee	500 Waukegan Road Deerfield, IL 60015 312/948-6138

Company/Division	Address/Phone #
Schwartau of America	111 Barclay Boulevard Lincolnshire, IL 60069 312/634-8280
Scott Paper Company	Scott Plaza II Philadelphia, PA 19113 215/522-6760
The Seven-Up Company	121 S. Meramec St. Louis, MO 63105 314/889-8050 or 426-8220
The J. M. Smucker Company	Strawberry Lane Orrville, OH 44667 216/682-0015 ext. 237
Sun Diamond Company	1050 S. Diamond Street Stockton, CA 95201 209/467-6000
Sunkist Growers, Inc.	616 E. Sunkist Street Ontario, CA 91761 714/983-9811 ext. 262
Tambrands, Inc.	P.O. Box 271 Palmer, MA 01069 413/283-3431

Company/Division	Address/Phone #
Tetley, Inc.	100 Commerce Drive Shelton, CT 06484 203/929-9311
Tropicana Products, Inc.	P.O. Box 338 Bradenton, FL 33506 813/747-4461
Uncle Ben's, Inc.	P.O. Box 1752 Houston, TX 77251-1752 713/674-9484
Union Carbide	39 Old Ridgebury Road Danbury, CT 06817 203/794-7438
Universal Foods Corp.	433 E. Michigan Milwaukee, WI 53201 414/347-3797 or 271-6755
Wm. Wrigley Jr. Company	410 N. Michigan Avenue Chicago, IL 60611 312/644-2121

Index